Rehabilitation with rTMS

Masahiro Abo • Wataru Kakuda

Rehabilitation with rTMS

Springer

Masahiro Abo
Department of Rehabilitation Medicine
The Jikei University School of Medicine
Tokyo, Japan

Wataru Kakuda
Department of Rehabilitation Medicine
The Jikei University School of Medicine
Tokyo, Japan

ISBN 978-3-319-20981-4 ISBN 978-3-319-20982-1 (eBook)
DOI 10.1007/978-3-319-20982-1

Library of Congress Control Number: 2015957197

Springer Cham Heidelberg New York Dordrecht London

Printed on acid-free paper

Springer International Publishing AG Switzerland is part of Springer Science+Business Media (www.springer.com)

Contents

Authors

Masahiro Abo, Professor & Chairman, Department of Rehabilitation Medicine, The Jikei University School of Medicine

Wataru Kakuda, Associate Professor, Department of Rehabilitation Medicine, The Jikei University School of Medicine

Nobuyuki Sasaki, Associate professor, Department of Rehabilitation Medicine, International University of Health and Welfare

Toru Takekawa, Department of Rehabilitation Medicine, The Jikei University School of Medicine

Ryo Momosaki, Department of Rehabilitation Medicine, The Jikei University School of Medicine

Naoki Yamada, Department of Rehabilitation Medicine, The Jikei University School of Medicine

Takatoshi Hara, Department of Rehabilitation Medicine, The Jikei University School of Medicine

Yasuhide Nakayama, Department of Rehabilitation Medicine, The Jikei University School of Medicine

Motoi Watanabe, Department of Rehabilitation Medicine, The Jikei University School of Medicine

Junichi Nishimura, Department of Rehabilitation, Shimizu Hospital, The Kyosaikai Medical Foundation

Takahiro Kondo, Department of Rehabilitation, Shimizu Hospital, The Kyosaikai Medical Foundation

Yusuke Haga, Department of Rehabilitation, Tokyo General Hospital, The Kenkoukai Medical Foundation

Yoshihide Ishizuka, Department of Rehabilitation, Tokyo General Hospital, The Kenkoukai Medical Foundation

Toru Kurosaki, Department of Rehabilitation, Nishi-Hiroshima Rehabilitation Hospital, The Houwakai Medical Corporation

Facilities Conducting rTMS Treatment as of November 1, 2014

The Jikei University Hospital (Minato-Ku, Tokyo)
The Jikei University Daisan Hospital (Komae, Tokyo)
Shimizu Hospital, The Kyosaikai Medical Foundation (Kurayoshi, Tottori)
Tokyo General Hospital, The Kenkoukai Medical Foundation (Nakano-Ku, Tokyo)
Nishi-Hiroshima Rehabilitation Hospital, The Houwakai Medical Corporation (Hiroshima, Hiroshima)
Kimura Hospital, The Jujinkai Medical Corporation (Sabae, Fukui)
Kyoto Ohara Memorial Hospital, The Koryokai Medical Corporation (Kyoto, Kyoto)
Hakodate Shintoshi Hospital, The Yushinkai Medical Association (Hakodate, Hokkaido)
Kousei Hospital, The Corporate Medical Association Rokushinkai (Kobe, Hyogo)
Izumi Memorial Hospital, The Izenkai (Adachi-Ku, Tokyo)
Shin-Yurigaoka General Hospital, The Sanseikai (Kawasaki, Kanagawa)

(Upper limb hemiparesis) (Aphasia) (Dysphagia) (Lower limb hemiparesis)

- Out of the 11 facilities mentioned above, the Jikei University Hospital and Shimizu Hospital treat "upper limb hemiparesis" and "aphasia."
- The Jikei University Daisan Hospital treats "upper limb hemiparesis," "aphasia," "dysphagia" and "lower limb hemiparesis."
- The other eight facilities only treat "upper limb hemiparesis."

Introduction

In 1998, while studying at the Karolinska Institutet, I was blessed with the opportunity to use a magnetic stimulation device. I was surprised at how easily cerebral cortex could be stimulated with this device, and I still remember, as if it had been yesterday, the "tremor of excitement" that I felt when imagining that some day this magnetic stimulation device would contribute to the development of new therapies in the field of rehabilitation. For the clinical application of magnetic stimulation therapy, I first repeatedly conducted basic experiments using rat models of brain injury and stopped these temporarily after gaining first insights. Then, aiming to challenge the notion accepted worldwide that neurological sequelae of stroke will not improve in the chronic stage, to help patients who suffer from the neurological sequelae of stroke, and to further develop rehabilitation medicine, I made a point of calling on Dr. Wataru Kakuda, one of the authors and editors of this book, to return from Stanford University, and eventually in April 2008 we began to conduct NEURO therapy.

In *Treatment Approaches for the Recovery of Fine Motor Functions of the Hand and Finger by Use of rTMS and Intensive Occupational Therapy – Latest Rehabilitation Methods for the Treatment of Post-stroke Upper Limb Hemiparesis* (Miwa-Shoten Ltd.), which was published in July 2010, we introduced "NEURO" (a treatment protocol using rTMS treatment in combination with intensive rehabilitation), which our department developed and promoted for the first time in the world. In particular, during the last few years this NEURO therapy has been widely featured in the media, such as on TV, and an unending stream of patients have visited our department. To date more than 3000 patients with neurological sequelae of stroke, not only from throughout Japan but also from abroad, have visited our outpatient department. As a result, the number of patients who have undergone NEURO therapy has increased rapidly, and as of October 2014, in total more than 2000 patients have received the therapy at 13 affiliated and collaborative hospitals throughout Japan.

This book is a practical guide on "rTMS treatment and rehabilitation for the treatment of neurological sequelae of stroke." We have found that rTMS in combination with rehabilitation is useful not only for the treatment of poststroke upper limb hemiparesis but also for the treatment of other neurological sequelae of stroke, namely, aphasia, dysphagia, and lower limb hemiparesis and have published many research papers on this topic in international journals. Research resulted in as many as 14 research papers on the use of rTMS for the treatment of the neurological sequelae of stroke that can be accessed on PubMed (from 2010 to October 2014). Thus, it is no exaggeration to say that this book was written based on clinical data obtained from cases that we were involved in ourselves.

Since magnetic stimulation devices are currently approved for testing and not as therapeutic equipment, magnetic stimulation therapies such as NEURO are conducted based on the approval of the ethics committee of each institution that we collaborate with. Until recently, it was recommended that the upper limit of magnetic stimulation pulses should be 5000 pulses per week. However, according to the "Recommendations for Transcranial Magnetic Stimulation (TMS)" by the Committee on Brain Stimulation Methods of the Japanese Society of Clinical Neurophysiology (JSCN) in the *Japanese Journal for Clinical Neurophysiology* Vol. 40, No. 1, 2012, the upper limit of magnetic stimulation should be up to 15,000 pulses per week. Accordingly, magnetic stimulation conducted as in the case of NEURO therapy, which involves low-frequency stimulation with 14,400 pulses per week, is within the range of the upper limit recommended by the JSCN.

Finally, I want to express my gratitude to all members of the 13 hospitals who have banded together in the same spirit and cooperated in this clinical project. I hope that this book will be used by patients who suffer from neurological sequelae of stroke and their families and will serve as a reference for TMS treatment, which is one of a number of approaches to therapeutic rehabilitation.

October, 2014 Masahiro Abo

Chapter 1
rTMS and Its Potential Use in Stroke Rehabilitation

1 The Principle Behind TMS

The first report on the application of transcranial magnetic stimulation (TMS) as a new cerebral cortex stimulation technique that can be used as an alternative to direct electrical stimulation in humans was published in *the Lancet* in 1985. Barker [1] succeeded in painless recording of motor evoked potentials (MEPs) from the muscles of the hand and finger by transcranially applying a magnetic field, generated by an electric current passing through a circular coil, over the primary motor area of the cerebral cortex.

TMS consists of the TMS device main unit and a stimulation coil that is connected thereto (p. 119). The stimulation parameters (e.g., frequency, intensity, train duration) are set on the TMS device main unit, and TMS is conducted by applying the stimulation coil to the surface of the skull. Recently, there are also TMS devices with a cooling system that prevent an increase in the temperature of the coil, thus enabling prolonged continuous stimulation.

The principle by which the cerebral cortex is stimulated by TMS is based on the famous Faraday's law on electromagnetic induction. As shown in Fig. 1.1, when an electric current flows within a circular coil, a magnetic field (magnetic flux) is generated perpendicular to the plane of the coil and reaches the cerebral cortex after passing through soft tissues and the skull. To generate such a magnetic field, it is important that the electric current flowing through the coil is not a steady-state current but constantly changes its velocity.

In fact, the more rapidly the electric current flows, the greater becomes the magnetic field that is generated. The magnetic field that reaches the cerebral cortex generates an eddy current that is perpendicular to this magnetic field, and thus parallel to the plane of the coil (skull). The direction of the eddy current that is generated here is opposite to the direction of the electric current that flows through the coil. This eddy current acts on interneurons (that flow parallel to the skull) located in the cerebral cortex, and eventually also affects neurons throughout the brain stem and

M. Abo, W. Kakuda, *Rehabilitation with rTMS*,
DOI 10.1007/978-3-319-20982-1_1

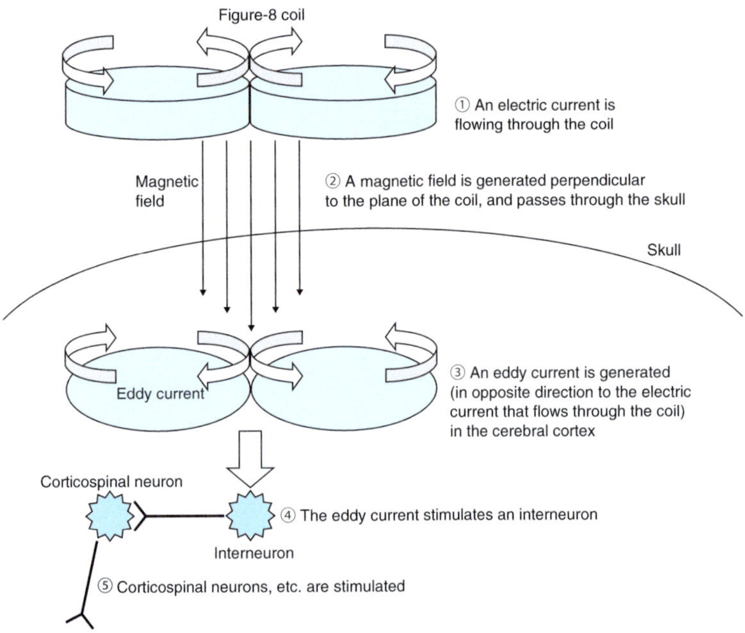

Fig. 1.1 Mechanism through which TMS stimulates the cerebral cortex

spinal cord that descend from the cerebral cortex. Thus, evidently TMS results in "transcranial" magnetic stimulation, but what actually affects the neurons is the eddy current that is generated in vivo by "magnetic stimulation."

The magnetic stimulation waves that are produced by TMS can be monophasic or biphasic waveforms. The biggest difference between these two kinds of waveforms is the number of neurons that are stimulated. More specifically, in the case of biphasic stimulation, which causes the electric current that flows through the coil to become bidirectional, more neurons are stimulated, and this stimulus reaches over a wider area than in case of monophasic stimulation. Regarding these differences, monophasic stimulation is considered appropriate for examinations in which MEPs, etc. are induced, and biphasic stimulation, which has a greater impact on the cerebral cortex, is considered to be more appropriate for therapeutic purposes such as described later.

The electric current that flows through the coil generates a magnetic field, which in turn generates an eddy current in vivo that flows in opposite direction to the electric current that is generated by the coil. Then interneurons are stimulated by this eddy current.

Schematic representation of the magnetic fields that are generated by these two types of stimulation coils (the higher the area is located, the greater is the magnetic field that is generated). While in the case of the circular coil the magnetic field at the center of the loop becomes almost zero (in this figure represented as "a hollow"), in case of the figure-8 coil the maximum magnetic field is in the center of the coil (at the intersection of the two loops) (in this figure represented as "a peak").

There are two types of TMS stimulation coils that are typically used, circular coils and figure-8 coils (Fig. 1.2). As shown in Fig. 1.3 there are differences in the distribution of the magnetic field that is generated by these two types of coils. First, when using a circular coil the highest magnetic field is generated beneath the coil loop, and the magnetic field beneath the center of the coil becomes zero. Therefore, circular coils are suitable for the indefinite stimulation of a wide area of the cerebral cortex; however, circular coils are by no means suitable for the local stimulation of narrow sites of the cerebral cortex, regardless of whether TMS is used for examinations or therapeutic purposes. In contrast, when using a figure-8 coil the two eddy currents that are generated by magnetic stimulation at the intersection of its two loops overlap, and the strongest magnetic field is generated locally. Therefore, when conducting TMS

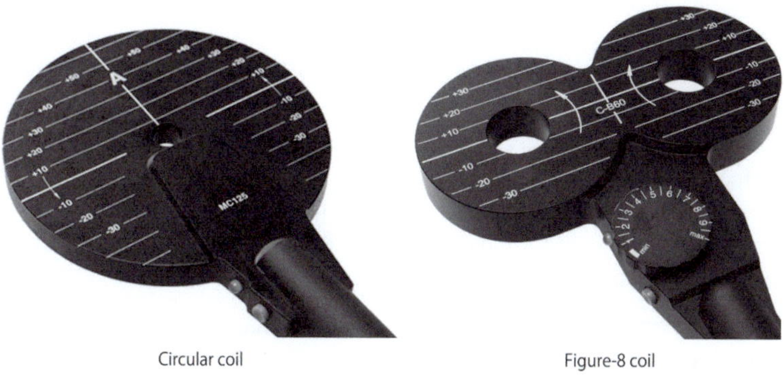

Fig. 1.2 Circular coil and figure-8 coil were both manufactured by MagVenture

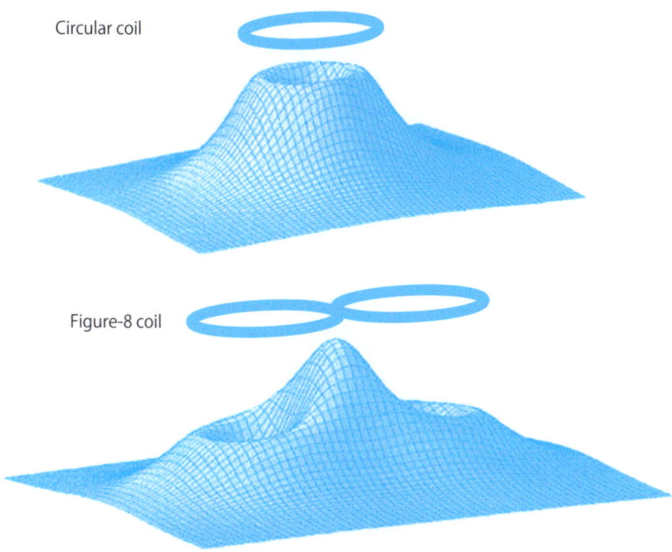

Fig. 1.3 Differences in the magnetic fields that are generated by these two types of coils

stimulation through which this intersection overlaps with the target area of the cerebral cortex, different from when using a circular coil, it becomes possible to stimulate an extremely limited area. Generally, the spatial resolution of figure-8 coils is considered to be within 5 mm, and at this intersection a magnetic force is generated that is several times higher than that at other sites of the coil. For this reason, at present TMS is considered an innovative device with which the cerebral cortex can be stimulated locally with high spatial resolution and without causing pain.

2 High-Frequency rTMS and Low-Frequency rTMS

As reported by Barker [1], initially TMS was used for physiological tests with the primary purpose to determine MEPs of peripheral muscles. However, hereafter with regard to repetitive transcranial magnetic stimulation (rTMS), it has been found that continuous application of TMS stimulation caused local changes to neural activity in the cortex. More specifically, it became clear that the application of rTMS stimulation affects brain "plasticity."

More specifically, besides the stimulation site, the following three factors serve as determinant parameters for the effect of rTMS on the cerebral cortex, and among these in particular the applied frequency plays an important role:

(i) Frequency of pulses (number of pulses per 1 second that are applied, expressed in Hz)
(ii) Intensity of pulses [expressed as the percentage (%) of the motor threshold (MT) (the minimum stimulus intensity that can induce muscle activity)]
(iii) Train duration (number of pulses that are applied)

This is because it has been confirmed that the effects of rTMS on the cerebral cortex greatly differ depending on the frequency of pulses. Generally, rTMS that is performed at a frequency of 5 Hz or higher is called high-frequency rTMS, and rTMS that is performed at a frequency of lower than 1 Hz is called low-frequency rTMS. However, in conclusion it has been found that while high-frequency rTMS enhances local neural activity of the stimulated site, low-frequency rTMS suppresses local neural activity at the stimulated site. Namely, the effects of rTMS on the cerebral cortex are completely opposite depending on the frequency used.

There are a number of reports that high-frequency rTMS enhances local neural activity of the cerebral cortex, including by Pascual-Leone et al. [2], who found that the amplitude of MEPs induced by primary motor area stimulation by use of the same stimulus intensity increased for approximately 3 minutes after applying a 10-pulse rTMS train at 20 Hz and 150 % of MT (train duration 0.5 seconds) to the primary motor area of the cerebral cortex (this was interpreted to mean that stimuli of the same intensity produced enhanced activity and excitability of the primary motor area of the cerebral cortex if they induced an increase in MEP amplitude). Similarly, Wu et al. [3] stated that the amplitude of MEP induced after applying a 30-pulse rTMS train at 15 Hz and 120 % MT (train duration 2 seconds) increased for 90 seconds. Moreover, an example in which stimuli below the motor threshold were used is, e.g., a report by Maeda et al. [4], who found that the size of MEP was amplified for 2 minutes after applying a 240-pulse rTMS train at 20 Hz and 90 % MT (train duration 12 seconds). They also pointed out that alteration of the local activity of the cerebral cortex with stimuli below the motor threshold requires prolonged stimulation.

In contrast, there are well-known reports, such as by Chen et al. [5] and Maeda et al. [6], that low-frequency rTMS suppresses local neural activity of the cerebral cortex. According to Chen et al. [5], after applying low-frequency rTMS, namely, a 810-pulse rTMS train at 0.9 Hz and 115 % of MT (train duration 15 minutes) to the primary motor area of the cerebral cortex, the MT of the stimulated side increased for 15 minutes and longer after stimulation (because it becomes difficult to receive a response to stimuli of the same intensity), and the amplitude of the induced MEPs decreased. Moreover, Maeda et al. [6] stated that MEPs decreased for 2 minutes when applying low-frequency rTMS, namely, a 240-pulse rTMS train at 1 Hz and 90 % of MT (train duration 4 minutes) only to one side of the primary motor area.

3 Neuromodulatory Mechanisms of rTMS

It is believed that the effects of rTMS on the local excitability of the cerebral cortex, more specifically, the mechanisms that underlie the neuromodulatory effects of rTMS, are alterations in synaptic efficiency (influence on synaptic signaling), which are the basis of brain plasticity. An increase in synaptic efficiency is called long-term potentiation (LTP), and a decrease in synaptic efficiency is called long-term depression (LTD). Conversely one can say that high-frequency rTMS induces LTP and low-frequency rTMS induces LTD.

According to the results of animal studies, LTP/LTD induction by rTMS appears to be mediated by neurotransmitters such as glutamate and gamma-aminobutyric acid (GABA). For instance, it has been confirmed in animal studies that inhibition of the glutamate-binding site on *N*-methyl-D-aspartate (NMDA) receptors by administrating NMDA receptor antagonists such as dextromethorphan or memantine reduces LTP/LTD induction resulting from rTMS [7, 8]. On the contrary, it has been reported that LTP/LTD induction resulting from rTMS is promoted when inhibiting inhibitory systems that are mediated by GABA [9]. This may be interpreted as meaning that while activation of the glutamate system enhances brain plasticity, activation of the GABA system decreases brain plasticity.

Since it has already been confirmed that brain plasticity is affected by various factors, it is conceivable that the degree of the neuromodulatory effect that is achieved by rTMS also undergoes similar effects. For instance, the blood levels of certain hormones appear to affect brain plasticity. Inghilleri et al. [10] examined the impact of the menstrual cycle on the effect of high-frequency rTMS in eight women. As a result, on Day 1 of the menstrual cycle no significant increase in the size of MEP was observed when applying high-frequency rTMS (5 Hz) to the primary motor area. However, on Day 14 of the menstrual cycle a significant increase in the size of MEP was observed when applying the same treatment. Based on this result, it was concluded that blood estrogen levels significantly affect the efficacy of high-frequency rTMS (along with increases in blood estrogen levels, brain plasticity, as well as the efficacy of rTMS increase).

Moreover, Sale et al. [11] investigated whether there are diurnal variations in the effects of paired-associative stimulation (PAS) consisting of peripheral nerve stimulation paired with rTMS on the primary motor area in 20 adults. As a result, a significant increase in the size of MEPs was observed both when PAS was conducted in the morning or afternoon, but the degree of increase was greater when PAS was conducted in the afternoon than when it was conducted in the morning. This result was interpreted to mean that there is a possibility that the blood levels of hormones that are closely related to the circadian rhythm such as melatonin and cortisol affect brain plasticity.

Moreover, brain plasticity has also been reported to be affected by certain genetic predispositions. After Kleim et al. [12] had suggested due to differences observed in the response to exercise therapy that brain-derived neurotrophic factor polymorphism (BDNF val66met polymorphism) affects brain plasticity, Cheeran et al. [13] examined the influence of BDNF polymorphisms on the effect of theta burst stimulation (TBS) (p. 164). When comparing the stimulatory and inhibitory effects of TBS in the group without the polymorphism [Val/Val type, where the nucleotides at codon 66 were both valine] and the group with the polymorphism [Val/Met type, where one of the nucleotides at codon 66 had mutated to methionine, or Met/Met type, where both nucleotides at codon 66 had mutated to methionine], it was found that in the group with polymorphism neither a sufficiently stimulatory nor inhibitory effect was exhibited, while in the group with no polymorphism significant changes were observed.

Therefore, for the therapeutic use of rTMS it is necessary to correctly identify under which circumstances brain plasticity increases, namely, whether the neuromodulatory effect of rTMS will be amplified or whether conversely plasticity will be reduced (namely, whether the effects of rTMS will be attenuated).

4 rTMS and Rehabilitation

It is believed that the so-called brain reorganization and restoration of impaired neuronal functions requires the functional and subsequent structural reorganization of the compensatory functional site as shown in Fig. 1.4, and the first step of this process can be interpreted as LTP/LTD induction.

For this reason the neuromodulatory effect of rTMS is undoubtedly expected to promote the "first step of brain reorganization." However, given the short duration of this effect, one can infer that the effect of rTMS is not sufficient to induce structural reorganization in a subsequent step. Accordingly, one can say for sure that rTMS increases brain plasticity; however, it is possible that the application of rTMS alone is not sufficient for achieving a long-lasting brain reorganization (in particular structural reorganization).

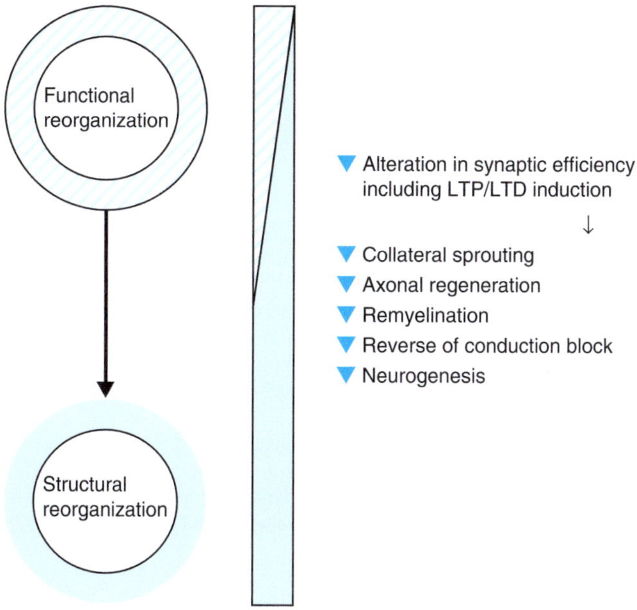

Fig. 1.4 Functional and structural reorganization in the restoration of neuronal functions. LTP/LTD induction is the first step of the reorganization of the brain when restoring neuronal function

Therefore, we thought that by combining rTMS with conventional rehabilitation it might be possible to clinically introduce rTMS as a therapeutic intervention for neurological sequelae of stroke that promotes the brain reorganization. In short, we thought that rTMS could take in the position of a preconditioning method that increases brain plasticity and that it would be optimal to combine rTMS with intensive rehabilitation. As a result, the concept of "rTMS and intensive rehabilitation combination therapy" described later became a fundamental idea that has yielded many favorable treatment outcomes. The combination of rTMS and intensive rehabilitation enhances the beneficial effect of each intervention procedure, and therefore this innovative therapy approach is increasingly used in clinical practice.

References

1. Barker AT. The history and basic principles of magnetic nerve stimulation. Electroencephalogr Clin Neurophysiol Suppl. 1999;51:3–21.
2. Pascual-Leone A, Valls-Solé J, Wassermann EM, et al. Responses to rapid-rate transcranial magnetic stimulation of the human motor cortex. Brain. 1994;117:847–58.
3. Wu T, Sommer M, Tergau F, et al. Lasting influence of repetitive transcranial magnetic stimulation on intracortical excitability in human subjects. Neurosci Lett. 2000;287:37–40.
4. Maeda F, Keenan JP, Tormos JM, et al. Interindividual variability of the modulatory effects of repetitive transcranial magnetic stimulation on cortical excitability. Exp Brain Res. 2000;133:425–30.

5. Chen R, Classen J, Gerloff C, et al. Depression of motor cortex excitability by low-frequency transcranial magnetic stimulation. Neurology. 1997;48:1398–403.
6. Maeda F, Keenan JP, Tormos JM, et al. Modulation of corticospinal excitability by repetitive transcranial magnetic stimulation. Clin Neurophysiol. 2000;111:800–5.
7. Stefan K, Kunesch E, Benecke R, et al. Mechanisms of enhancement of human motor cortex excitability induced by interventional paired associative stimulation. J Physiol. 2002;543:699–708.
8. Huang YZ, Chen RS, Rothwell JC, et al. The after-effect of human theta burst stimulation is NMDA receptor dependent. Clin Neurophysiol. 2007;118:1028–32.
9. Ziemann U, Hallett M, Cohen LG. Mechanisms of deafferentation-induced plasticity in human motor cortex. J Neurosci. 1998;18:7000–7.
10. Inghilleri M, Conte A, Currà A, et al. Ovarian hormones and cortical excitability. An rTMS study in humans. Clin Neurophysiol. 2004;115:1063–8.
11. Sale MV, Ridding MC, Nordstrom MA. Factors influencing the magnitude and reproducibility of corticomotor excitability changes induced by paired associative stimulation. Exp Brain Res. 2007;181:615–26.
12. Kleim JA, Chan S, Pringle E, et al. BDNF val66met polymorphism is associated with modified experience-dependent plasticity in human motor cortex. Nat Neurosci. 2006;9:735–7.
13. Cheeran B, Talelli P, Mori F, et al. A common polymorphism in the brain-derived neurotrophic factor gene (BDNF) modulates human cortical plasticity and the response to rTMS. J Physiol. 2008;586:5717–25.

Chapter 2
rTMS for Upper Limb Hemiparesis after Stroke

1 Pathology and Current Status of the Treatment

A. Current Status of Rehabilitation in Poststroke Upper Limb Hemiparesis

The mortality rate from stroke has been declining with the development of drug therapies in the acute phase and the established EBM for the treatment. Referring to the details of the "Japanese Guidelines for the Management of Stroke 2009," a rehabilitative intervention from the early stage after stroke onset is recommended as "Grade A" in the item of rehabilitation of motor disorders and activities of daily living (ADL) disability. Therefore, it is considered essential to perform consistent rehabilitation from the acute phase in stroke treatment (Table 2.1) [1]. However, in rehabilitation for motor disorders and ADL, facilitations (neuromuscular facilitation procedures) [including the Bobath method, neurodevelopmental exercise (Davis), proprioceptive neuromuscular facilitation (PNF) method, and the Brunnstrom method] are classified as Grade C. In addition, in the item of rehabilitation of upper limb dysfunction in the guidelines, repetitive motion exercise, goal-oriented exercise, and constraint-induced movement (CI) therapy, which suppresses the movement of the unaffected upper limb, are considered useful, as shown in Table 2.2 [1]. These facts have been demonstrated also in the rehabilitation of post-stroke upper limb hemiparesis published in the Lancet, described below [2].

B. Functional Recovery of Poststroke Upper Limb Hemiparesis

As described above, it is considered that the number of patients with severe upper limb hemiparesis has been declining with the introduction of rehabilitation from the acute phase. However, relatively few stroke patients became able to use their

M. Abo, W. Kakuda, *Rehabilitation with rTMS*,
DOI 10.1007/978-3-319-20982-1_2

Table 2.1 Rehabilitation of motor disorders and ADL

1. For neurological sequelae of stroke, it is strongly recommended to actively perform rehabilitation from an early stage in order to facilitate the recovery of dysfunction and decreased function (Grade A)
2. For patients in the early stage after stroke onset, it is recommended to increase the frequency and amount of training in order to facilitate the recovery of decreased function more effectively (Grade A)
3. Facilitations (neuromuscular facilitation procedures) [including Bobath method, neurodevelopmental exercise (Davis), proprioceptive neuro-muscular facilitation (PNF) method and Brunnstrom method] can be performed; however, there is no scientific evidence that shows these methods are more effective than traditional rehabilitation (Grade C1)

Excerpt from Ref. [1]

Table 2.2 Rehabilitation of upper limb dysfunction

1. For the upper limb on the paralyzed side, it is strongly recommended to actively repeat a specific training (including reach exercise of the upper limb on the paralyzed side, repetitive exercise of both upper limbs along with a metronome, goal-oriented exercise, and image training) (Grade A)
2. For patients with mild paralysis, it is recommended to administer a treatment by suppressing the movement of the upper limb on the non-paralyzed side and forcing the patient to use the upper limb on the paralyzed side in daily life, provide d that the indication is properly selected (Grade B)
3. For moderately paralyzed muscles, in particular for strengthening the wrist dorsiflexor muscle, electrical stimulation is recommended (Grade B)

Reprinted from Ref. [1]

paralyzed upper limb as a functional hand after rehabilitation. In a previous report on the functional prognosis in patients with poststroke upper limb hemiparesis, Duncan et al. [3] reported that significant improvement can be observed within 1 month of the stroke onset and most patients reach a plateau state by 6 months after the stroke onset (Fig. 2.1). In addition, Jorgensen et al. [4] reported that patients with mild, moderate, and severe upper limb hemiparesis reach a plateau state in 6 weeks, 10 weeks, and 15 weeks after the stroke onset, respectively. Most patients with poststroke upper limb hemiparesis undergo an evaluation of the functional prognosis of their paralyzed hand, based on which they receive rehabilitation to acquire the ADL necessary for them. For example, patients with mild paralysis mainly receive dexterity training such as chopsticks operation, handwriting, and cup retention.

In moderate to severe cases, a patient changes hand dominance or performs using one hand movements that had previously been performed with both hands. In other words, a "compensatory approach" is generally adopted in many cases in the general rehabilitation from the recovery to maintenance phase.

However, findings on poststroke cerebral plasticity in recent years show that there is some plasticity even in the chronic stage of stroke patients after some time has elapsed from the onset. For example, CI therapy, which intensively approaches

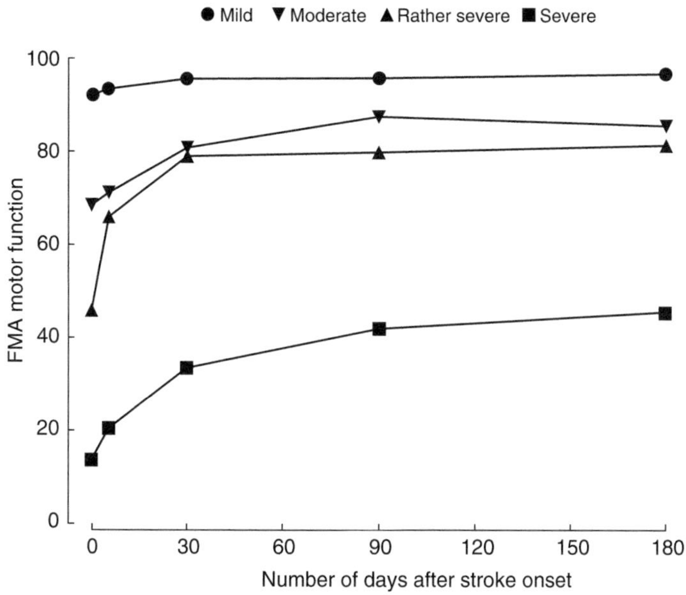

Fig. 2.1 Changes in post-stroke upper limb hemiparesis score. After the stroke onset, the FMA score of upper limb hemiparesis reaches a plateau state on Day 90 regardless of the severity (Adopted from Ref. [3])

the upper limb on the paralyzed side, is one of the neurorehabilitations (hereinafter, NR) widely performed in chronic stroke patients. Previous reports on brain functional reorganization in CI therapy indicated that improvement of the upper limb on the paralyzed side is related to the expansion of the neural plastic area of the lesional hemisphere and that it could influence on the interhemispheric balance [5, 6]. Thus, it is now considered that there is a possibility of maximizing the upper limb function by influencing the cerebral plasticity even in patients with poststroke upper limb hemiparesis who were previously believed to have reached a functional plateau. In this context, another type of "rehabilitation approach for functional recovery" is beginning to attract attention.

In the systematic review of poststroke rehabilitation published by Langhorne et al. [2] in 2009, the results of randomized controlled trials (RCTs) of rehabilitation training for a variety of strokes in the past were statistically analyzed. According to this report, 88 studies (total of 2687 patients) of upper limb training and 37 studies (total of 1467 patients) of hand-finger training were identified. In the upper limb training, CI therapy, myoelectric feedback, electrical stimulation therapy, and robot training are reported to be highly effective. On the other hand, in finger training, the results showed that a sufficient effect cannot be obtained even after the same training as that for upper limb cases was performed. Under these circumstances, repetitive transcranial magnetic stimulation (rTMS) has recently started attracting attention as an NR method.

C. Current Status of rTMS

rTMS is an up-and-coming treatment method, which is applied to bring out the potential of the brain reorganization by directly stimulating the cerebral cortex. As an EBM for rTMS, a meta-analysis of rTMS treatment for stroke patients was reported in 2012 [7].

In this report, 18 articles published from 2005 through 2011 were reviewed (in 5 of the articles, two stimulation approaches were applied), where rTMS was performed in a total of 392 patients. Looking at the details, they varied in terms of the time from the onset to the intervention. Three articles focused on the acute phase, another three focused on the subacute phase, seven articles focused on the chronic phase, and the remaining articles dealt with various phases. With respect to the lesions, 6 articles covered subcortical lesions, and 11 articles covered both subcortical and cortical lesions (the remaining 1 article compared subcortical and cortical lesions). With respect to the stimulation method, the following methods were applied: a low-frequency rTMS to the unaffected hemisphere in eight studies, a high-frequency rTMS to the affected hemisphere in five studies, a low-frequency rTMS to the affected hemisphere in one study, both low-frequency rTMS to the unaffected hemisphere and high-frequency rTMS to the affected hemisphere in two studies, and theta burst stimulation (TBS) (p. 164) in the remaining two studies.

Of the 392 patients studied in 18 articles, adverse effects were observed in 4 patients, in whom headache and fatigue occurred, but no serious convulsive seizure was reported. As a consequence, the effect size was 0.55 when all the articles were collectively analyzed. When comparing the low-frequency and the high-frequency rTMS in the subgroup analysis, the effect size was 0.69 and 0.41, respectively, which means that low-frequency rTMS is superior. According to the lesions, the results showed that the effect size of subcortical lesions was 0.73 and that of the other lesions was 0.45. That is, rTMS is more effective in patients with subcortical lesions.

From these results, rTMS is believed to bring significant improvements in post-stroke upper limb hemiparesis and is expected to produce a greater effect through performing the treatment in accordance with the stimulation method, lesions, and intervention time.

Thus, we found that rTMS is effective for poststroke upper limb hemiparesis and particularly significant effects can be obtained when low-frequency rTMS is performed on the unaffected hemisphere during the chronic phase. The detailed protocol and treatment outcome of our ongoing study, "NEURO-15 (NovEl intervention Using Repetitive TMS and intensive Occupational therapy-15 days protocol)," will be described below. This protocol began to be implemented in April 2009 after a process of trial and error, and ongoing studies are being carried out based on the same philosophy and protocol at nine institutions throughout Japan. The total number of patients receiving NEURO was more than 2000 as of October 2014. Not only the number of patients who experienced the therapy but also results as well are unprecedented in Japan.

2 Protocol of the Combination Treatment of Low-Frequency rTMS and Intensive Occupational Therapy

A. Overview of NEURO-15

1) Eligibility Criteria

The major eligibility criteria of NEURO-15 are set as shown in Table 2.3, based on not only the contraindications and precautions published in the previous guidelines of rTMS treatment that Wassermann [8] proposed (Wassermann Guidelines) but also the eligibility criteria of CI therapy [9] which have been traditionally proposed. Today, these are used as common criteria for all institutions.

2) Details of rTMS Treatment

Low-frequency rTMS is applied using MagPro R30 and a figure-8 coil (both are manufactured by Magventure A/S). The stimulation site for low-frequency rTMS is the primary motor hand and finger area of the nonlesional hemisphere; that is, the optimal site of stimulation defined as the location where the largest motor evoked potentials (MEPs) in the first dorsal interosseous (FDI) muscle of the unaffected upper limb was elicited on electromyography (Fig. 2.2). The intensity of stimulation is set at 90 % of the motor threshold (the minimum stimulus intensity that can produce MEP at the stimulation site), and a low-frequency rTMS of 1 Hz is applied to the unaffected hemisphere for 20 minutes (a total of 1200 pulses) per session (Table 2.4). In principle, the patient must be attended by a physician during

Table 2.3 Eligibility criteria of NEURO-15

1. BRS for hand-fingers on the paralyzed side of 3–5. (At least, the hand and finger can be actively flexed without any problems. However it does not matter whether or not the patient can perform isolated movement when determining eligibility)
2. Age (at the time of determining the eligibility) between 18 and 90 years
3. Time between onset and intervention of more than 12 months
4. History of a single stroke only (no bilateral cerebrovascular lesion)
5. No significant cognitive impairment (preferably a Mini Mental State Examination score of more than 26)
6. No active systemic or mental illness requiring medical management
7. No recent history of seizure for at least one year preceding the intervention
8. No abnormal wave form, such as epileptic discharge on electroencephalogram (electroencephalogram as a screening test is performed only in patients with a history of seizures and in patients receiving an oral anti-epileptic drug)
9. No contraindications listed in the guidelines proposed by Wassermann (such as the presence of intracranial metal objects, the presence of a cardiac pacemaker, and pregnancy)

As of December 2012

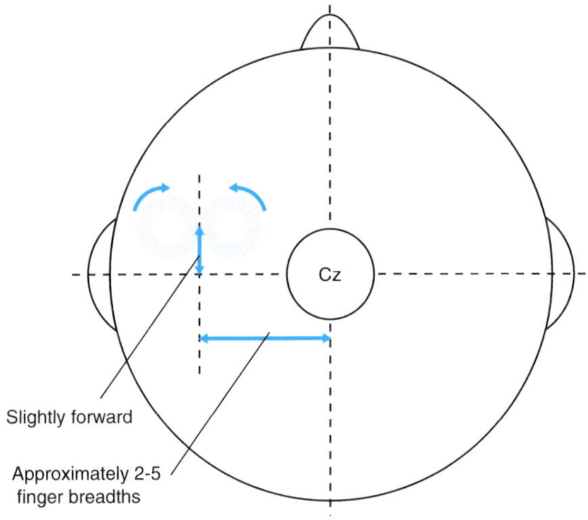

Fig. 2.2 Stimulation site for low frequency rTMS. Stimulate the motor center for the hand and finger which is located about 2–5 finger breadths away from Cz (vertex) based on the international 10–20 method, and slightly forward

Table 2.4 An example of rTMS treatment in NEURO-15[a]

Coil used	Figure-8 coil
Site	Non-lesional hemisphere (prim. motor hand and finger area)
Intensity	90 % of motor threshold
Frequency	Low-frequency rTMS (1 Hz)
Duration	1 session lasting 20 minutes (1200 pulses), once or twice daily
Days in hosp.	15 days

[a]The actual treatment is adjusted by each institution (As of December 2012)

stimulation. As a matter of our policy, the treatment should be immediately discontinued when adverse events (e.g., convulsion, headache, and discomfort of stimulation site) or other neurological symptoms occur.

3) Treatment Schedule

NEURO-15 is a therapeutic intervention that is performed during hospitalization, in principle. Table 2.5 shows an example of a training schedule during hospitalization. Over the course of a 15-day hospitalization, a treatment session consisting of low-frequency rTMS over the nonlesional hemisphere and intensive occupational therapy (OT) is performed twice daily in principle (except Sundays). Prior to applying NEURO-15, we make it a rule to obtain the consent of each study patient after providing them with sufficient information about the treatment.

Table 2.5 An example hospitalization schedule of NEURO-15[a]

Fri.	Saturday	Sun.	Monday to Saturday	Sun.	Monday-Tuesday	Wednesday
Evaluation at admission	Low-frequency rTMS (20 minutes)	No treatment	Low-frequency rTMS (20 minutes)	No treatment	Low-frequency rTMS (20 minutes)	
	One-to-one training (60 minutes)		One-to-one training (60 minutes)		One-to-one training (60 minutes)	
	Self-exercise (60 minutes)		Self-exercise (60 minutes)		Self-exercise (60 minutes)	
Low-frequency rTMS (20 minutes)			Low-frequency rTMS (20 minutes)		Low-frequency rTMS (20 minutes)	Evaluation at discharge
One-to-one training (60 minutes)			One-to-one training (60 minutes)		One-to-one training (60 minutes)	
Self-exercise (60 minutes)			Self-exercise (60 minutes)		Self-exercise (60 minutes)	

[a]An example of being hospitalized on a Thursday. The actual hospitalization schedule is adjusted by each institution (As of December 2012)

B. OT Evaluation in NEURO-15

At the time of admission and discharge, (1) the upper limb function on the paralyzed side and (2) the usage of the paralyzed side in daily life are evaluated.

1) Evaluation of Upper Limb Function

The evaluations of upper limb function conducted in NEURO-15 are as follows:

(i) Brunnstrom recovery stage (BRS)
(ii) Ueda's 12-grade motor function test for hemiplegia
(iii) Fugl-Meyer assessment (FMA)
(iv) Wolf motor function test (WMFT)
(v) Modified Ashworth scale (MAS)
(vi) Simple test for evaluating hand function (STEF)
(vii) Ten second test
(viii) Grip strength
(ix) Range of motion (ROM)
(x) Sensory examination
(xi) Action research arm test (ARAT)

BRS is a method to clinically classify the recovery process of paralysis caused by central nervous system injury by focusing on synergies (Table 2.6) [10]. It is classified into six stages from I to VI, which qualitatively evaluate a series of recovery processes: first, the flaccid state in the acute phase is observed, associative reactions and synergies appear, individual movements can be observed, and normal movements gradually return with the attenuation of spasticity. However, patients with paralysis do not uniformly follow this recovery process and may stop recovering at a certain stage according to the lesion. In Japan, BRS is widely used as the most basic and common qualitative functional evaluation method of central motor paralysis. However, it has some disadvantages: the range varies by each stage, and the stages are not classified in a detailed manner. Thus, this is mainly used as a screening tool.

FMA is a scale suitable to comprehensively evaluate the recovery of motor function. It enables us not only to determine the motor function of the upper and lower limbs by focusing on the synergy pattern but also to evaluate the balance, sensation, ROM, and other aspects (Table 2.7) [11]. In the study patients of NEURO-15, we use 33 items selected from FMA, which are related to the upper limb function such

Table 2.6 Brunnstrom recovery stage (upper limb, hand and finger)

Stage	Upper limb	Hand and finger
I	Flaccid. No voluntary movement	Flaccid
II	Voluntary elevation, retraction, abduction, external rotation, and extension of the shoulder, and voluntary flexion and supination of the elbow can be slightly or partly observed	Voluntary finger flexion is almost impossible
III	(a) Volitional flexion within synergies described in Stage II can be partly done voluntarily (b) In addition, volitional extension within synergies, including depression, protrusion, adduction, internal rotation and flexion of the shoulder, and extension and pronation of the elbow can be done voluntarily	Mass flexion can be done, but mass extension cannot be done Voluntary finger extension cannot be done, but reflexive extension can be done
IV	(a) Can stretch the arm forward (b) Can pronate and supinate with keeping the elbow close to the side and flexing it at 90 degrees (c) Can roll the arm back and touch the waist	A lateral side pinch can be done and release by moving the thumb also can be done Voluntary finger flexion can be done slightly
V	(a) Can stretch the arm forward and elevate it higher than Stage IV (b) Can stretch the arm to the side (c) Can pronate and supinate the forearm with the elbow at the extended position	Finger grip, cylinder grip and ball grip can be done. Can spread all the fingers and the thumb
VI	Can perform the isolated movements described in Stage V quickly, easily and coordinately Normal movements returned or almost returned	All kinds of grips can be done well. Voluntary finger extension can be done over the entire range of motion Individual movements of the finger also can be done

Reprinted from Ref. [10]

Table 2.7 Fugl-Meyer assessment [1. Motor function and balance (upper limb)]

Evaluation item				Score		
AA shoulder/elbow/forearm (subtotal/36 points)				None	Sufficient	Insufficient
I. Reflex		Biceps and finger flexor		0		2
		Triceps		0		2
II. Volitional movement within synergies	(a) Flexor[a]	Shoulder	Retraction		1	2
			Elevation	0	1	2
			Abduction	0	1	2:>90°
			External rotation	0	1	2
		Elbow	Flexion		1	2
		Forearm	Supination	0	1	2
	(b) Extensor[b]	Shoulder	Adduction/internal rotation	0	1	2
		Elbow	Extension		1	2
		Forearm	Pronation	0	1	2
III. Volitional movement mixing synergies (flexor/extensor)		Move the arm around to the lumbar spine in a sitting posture		0	1: Just beyond anterior superior iliac spine	2
		Shoulder flexion at 90° with elbow in an extended position and the forearm in an intermediary position		0	1: The elbow flexes at a later stage	2
		Pronation and supination with the shoulder at 0° and the elbow flexed at 90°		0	1	2

(continued)

Table 2.7 (continued)

Evaluation item		Score		
IV. Volitional movement with little or no synergies	Shoulder abduction at 90° with elbow at an extended position and forearm at a pronated position in a sitting posture	0	1: The elbow flexes and the forearm supinates during the process	2
	Shoulder flexion at 180° with the elbow at an extended position	0	1: The elbow flexes at a later stage	2
	Pronation and supination with elbow at an extended position and with shoulder at a flexed position at 30 to 90°	0	1	2
V. Normal reflex activity[c]	Examine the tendon jerks of I	0	1: >1 increased reflex response, >2 mild increased reflex responses	2
B. Wrist joint[d] (subtotal/10 points)		None	Sufficient	Insufficient
Keep the dorsiflexion in the wrist joint at 15° with the shoulder at 0° and the elbow flexion at 90°		0	1: Can be performed if no resistance is applied	2: Can be performed even if gentle resistance is applied
Volar flexion/dorsiflexion in the wrist joint		0	1	2: Can be performed over the whole range of motion
With the shoulder in a slightly flexed and abducted position the elbow in an extended position, and the forearm in a pronated position	Keep the dorsiflexion in the wrist joint at 15°		1: Can be performed if no resistance is applied	2: Can be performed even if gentle resistance is applied
	Repeated volar flexion/dorsiflexion in the wrist joint	0	1	2: Can be performed over the whole range of motion
	Circumduction	0	1	2: Can be smoothly performed and have sufficient range of motion
C. Finger[e] (subtotal/14 points)		None	Sufficient	Insufficient
Mass flexion		0	1	2
Mass extension		0	1	2
Grasp	(a) Digit 2–5 extension in MCP, flexion in PIP and DIP	0	1: Weak	2: Can be performed even if strong resistance is applied

	(b) Pinch a piece of paper using the index finger's MP joint and the thumb at the extended position	0	1: The paper can be pulled out by weak force	2: The paper cannot be pulled out
	(c) Pinch a pencil using the pads of the thumb and the index finger	0	1: The paper can be pulled out by weak force	2: The paper cannot be pulled out
	(d) Cylinder grip	0	1: The paper can be pulled out by weak force	2: The paper cannot be pulled out
	(e) Grip a tennis ball with the thumb at the opposed position	0	1: The paper can be pulled out by weak force	2: The paper cannot be pulled out
D. Coordination/speed[f] (subtotal/6 points)		None	Sufficient	Insufficient
Tremor		0 : Noticeable	1 : mild	2 : None
Dysmetria		0: Noticeable	1 : mild	2 : None
Time		0 : >6 seconds	1 : 2–5 seconds	2 : <2 seconds
Total score			// 66 points	

[a]Lift the hand up to the ear on the paralyzed side in a sitting position
[b]Touch the knee on the non-paralyzed side in a sitting position
[c]This test should be performed only when a patient achieves a perfect score in IV
[d]Give assistance to keep the position of the shoulder and the arm if needed (Adopted from Ref. [11])
[e]Give assistance to keep the arm at 90 degrees if needed
[f]Repeat the movement of putting the index finger on the paralyzed side to the nose five times as fast as possible with eyes closed (Adopted from Ref. [11])

as the forearm's pronation and supination and the elbow joint's extension. Each item is rated on a three-point ordinal scale: 0 point (cannot), 1 point (can perform partially), and 2 points (can perform fully). This means that the maximum motor performance score for the upper limb that can be attained is 66 points.

WMFT is an objective evaluation method that was created to evaluate the function of the upper limb on the paralyzed side before and after CI therapy. It has come to be used more frequently, especially in Western countries. It consists of 15 tasks (6 physical exercises and 9 object manipulations), and the required time for completing each task is measured and recorded. Each task should be completed within 120 seconds. When the task was not completed within 120 seconds, the performance time of the task was recorded as 120 seconds. Eventually, the total performance time (seconds) of all 15 tasks or the natural logarithm of the average performance time are considered as an evaluated value. The smaller this value is, the better the upper limb function is. In addition, the quality of movement is determined on a six-level rating system in the functional ability scale (FAS), from 0 (cannot move at all) to 5 (can move almost normally).

ARAT is not very common in Japan. However, some reports indicate that it has high reliability and validity as an evaluation method of poststroke upper limb function [12, 13] and it is widely used in the United States and Europe. It was developed based on the upper extremity function test (UEFT) [14] by Lyle [15] to assess the poststroke upper limb function. UEFT was developed to monitor the upper limb functions related to daily life and consists of 33 evaluation items in total. In ARAT, the 4 major functions of upper limbs, that is, (1) grab, (2) grasp, (3) pinch, and (4) gross motor, were selected from the evaluation items of UEFT and organized into 19 items in total. ARAT's features are as follows: it is relatively simple and easy to use because the evaluation requires only a mean of 5 to 10 minutes, gross motor-related subtests are included in the items, and its score can be widely distributed even in cases of severe paralysis.

2) Evaluation of Use in Daily Life

We make an evaluation of the amount of use (AOU) which subjectively shows how often the upper limb on the paralyzed side is used in daily life as well as the quality of movement (QOM), which shows how well it is used. In fact, there are few scales to evaluate the severity of upper limb paralysis from the point of view of the ADL and instrumental activity of daily living (IADL). Therefore, evaluation is made by using (1) a Japanese version of MAL (Tables 2.8 and 2.9) prepared by Takahashi et al. [16] through summarizing a motor activity log (MAL) that has already been put to practical use and (2) a Jikei assessment scale for motor impairment in daily living (JASMID) (Tables 2.10 and 2.11) devised by Ishikawa et al. in our department [17].

MAL comprises 14 ADL items that were devised based on the Western lifestyle and has come to be used more frequently, mainly in the United States.

Table 2.8 Japanese version of motor activity log

Motion evaluation items	AOU	QOM
1. Read a book/newspaper/magazine while holding it		
2. Wipe my face and body with a towel		
3. Pick up a glass		
4. Brush my teeth with a toothbrush		
5. Put on makeup/shave		
6. Open a door by using a key		
7. Write a letter/type		
8. Stand still in a stable position		
9. Put my arm through the sleeve		
10. Move an object with my hand		
11. Eat by holding a fork or a spoon		
12. Comb hair by using a brush or a comb		
13. Hold a cup by grasping its handle		
14. Fasten the front buttons		
Total		
Mean (total/number of motion evaluation items which have been performed)		

Reprinted from Ref. [16]

Table 2.9 Evaluation scale for Japanese version of motor activity log

AOU (amount of use)
0. Do not use my weaker arm (not used; 0 % of pre-stroke)
1. Occasionally use my weaker arm, but only very rarely (very rarely used; 5 % of pre-stroke)
2. Sometimes use my weaker arm but do the activity most of the time only with my stronger arm (rarely used; 25 % of pre-stroke)
3. Use my weaker arm about half as often as before the stroke (50 % of pre-stroke).
4. Use my weaker arm almost as often as before the stroke (75 % of pre-stroke).
5. Use my weaker arm as often as before the stroke (100 % of pre-stroke)
QOM (quality of movement)
0. My weaker arm is not used at all (not used)
1. My weaker arm is moved during the activity but is not helpful (very poor)
2. My weaker arm is of some use during the activity but needs some help from the stronger arm, moves very slowly, or with difficulty (poor)
3. My weaker arm is used for the activity but the movements are slow or it is not strong enough (fair)
4. The movements made by my weaker arm for the activity are almost normal but not quite as fast or accurate as normal (almost normal)
5. The ability to use my weaker arm for the activity is as good as before the stroke (normal)

Adapted from Ref. [16]

Table 2.10 JASMID

Motion evaluation items[a]	AOU	QOM
1. Write with a pen[b]		
2. Eat with chopsticks (pick up side dishes)[b]		
3. Brush my teeth with a toothbrush[c]		
4. Clip the fingernails		
5. Open and hold an umbrella		
6. Put on makeup/shave[c]		
7. Wash my face		
8. Comb hair by using a brush or a comb		
9. Fasten the front buttons of a shirt[d]		
10. Turn a page of a newspaper/a magazine and read it[d]		
11. Open and close the lid of a plastic bottle[d]		
12. Cut toilet paper roll[d]		
13. Open a can of juice[d]		
14. Fasten a belt/put on a brassiere[d]		
15. Put on socks (for both feet)		
16. Wring out a rag or a towel		
17. Hang up a jacket on a hanger		
18. Take some coins out of a purse		
19. Tie shoelaces		
20. Wear a tie/necklace		
Engage in hobbies		
Engage in work/do housework		
Total		

Reprinted from Ref. [17]
[a]Regardless of the use of self-help tools such as an electric toothbrush and chopsticks with handles
[b]For motion evaluation items 1 and 2, motions as a "supporting hand" are excluded
[c]For motion evaluation items 3 and 6, preparing motions are not evaluated
[d]For motion evaluation items 9–14, motions as a "supporting hand" are also included

On the other hand, JASMID was examined and developed to solve the problems of adapting MAL directly to patients in Japan. It is a scale to evaluate the severity of upper limb paralysis from the point of view of ADL and IADL in line with the Japanese lifestyle. We are working toward practical use of JASMID.

C. Intensive OT in NEURO-15

1) Concept

NEURO-15's goal is for patients to acquire a habit of using the upper limb on the paralyzed side (as much as possible) also in daily life after discharge when they need.

Table 2.11 Evaluation scale and scoring system of JASMID

AOU (amount of use)
0. Do not use my weaker arm at all (do not want to use it)
1. Cannot use my weaker arm at all (want to use it but cannot)
2. Use my weaker arm a little (rarely use it)
3. Sometimes use my weaker arm (only 50 % of pre-stroke)
4. Often use my weaker arm (use it less frequently than pre-stroke)
5. Always use my weaker arm (use it as often as pre-stroke)
QOM (quality of movement)
0. Can rarely use my weaker arm (even if try to do it)
1. Find it very difficult to use my weaker arm (quite difficult compared to pre-stroke)
2. Find it moderately difficult to use my weaker arm (50 % of difficulty compared to pre-stroke)
3. Find it slightly difficult to use my weaker arm (slight difficulty compared to pre-stroke)
4. Do not find it difficult to use my weaker arm at all (almost the same as pre-stroke)
Scoring system
Frequency of use = sum of AOU/(number of motion items scored at 1 to 4 × 5) × 100
Quality of movement = sum of QOM/(number of answered motion items × 5) × 100

Reprinted from Ref. [17]

Most patients who have received NEURO-15 said as follows: "I cannot imagine moving my weaker upper limb," "I don't know how to move it," or "I've forgotten how to use it." We attribute this to the fact that most patients have fallen into a motion pattern specific to chronic stroke hemiplegia (a situation where labored movements are repeated because of the central hypotonia and this causes muscle tone in the peripheral portion to increase, which inhibits isolated movements).

We therefore believe that it is necessary to assess the states of motor paralysis through a comprehensive evaluation, as follows: (1) it is functionally impossible for the patient to do it; (2) the patient has not learned how to use it, although he/she has a function that can be used; or (3) as a result of prioritizing work efficiency when using the nonparalyzed upper limb, the patient has learned not to use it (learned nonuse) and does not use it even if he/she can.

In any case, we have made interventions in consideration of the fact that most patients have fallen into a situation where there are less opportunities to use their fingers on the paralyzed side as a result that the paralyzed upper limb has rarely been used and the nonparalyzed upper limb has mainly been used in daily life over a long period of time.

2) Point of the Program Structure

In the NR, the major functional recovery process from the subacute to chronic phase is considered as a reorganization of the neural mechanism in a usage frequency-dependent manner. Therefore, it is considered that the volume of training, training time, training content, and environment, including task-oriented movements, are important for performing the NR efficiently and effectively and that rebuilding the brain function can be promoted, especially by increasing the volume of task-oriented training [18, 19].

NEURO-15 has been implemented as a 15-day rehabilitation program, including about 4 hours intensive OT daily. This means that it includes sufficient training time, as described above. In addition, its short-term program aims to acquire a patient's needs after fully understanding his/her functional capacity. To achieve this goal, it consists of step-by-step programs that aim to acquire the movements that the patient needs most and that will probably be used more often in his/her daily life, such as those for ADL and hobbies. It is safe to say that this is task-oriented training.

If we conclude that it is very hard to get the patient to achieve his/her needs, the therapist may make a proposal to perform training including movements considered acquirable. In any case, it is important to carry out interventions that can improve the quality of life after discharge. And it is necessary to prepare a self-exercise program suitable for each patient based on the goal of continuing to use the upper limb on the paralyzed side.

D. Actual Practice of Intensive OT in NEURO-15

1) Questionnaire Before Admission

Our department conducts a survey using a questionnaire (by mail) prior to admission and makes an effort to understand the patient's requests and needs about the treatment and his/her use of the upper limb on the paralyzed side in daily life. By referring to the survey results, we provide an individual OT program with an emphasis on meeting the patient's needs.

2) One-to-One OT

Considering the clinical presentations of the study patients in NEURO-15 described so far, if an occupational therapist asks a patient to move only the distal portion without fully considering the motor disorder of the central portion, the stability and individuality of movements were ignored, resulting in gross motor movement without dexterity and simply causing patients to "overstrain" themselves. In other words, if a patient trains the upper limb on the paralyzed side in his/her own way, there is a risk that it would end up learning the incorrect movements with the result that a desirable recovery would not be achieved. For this reason, it is especially important to conduct iterative training with facilitation procedures and provide practical ADL and IADL training with direct intervention of an occupational therapist.

We basically start our individual OT in a hands-on manner and provide a patient with "infallible learning" and make an intervention for efficient motor learning.

Then, while observing the patient's motion patterns and his/her status of motion acquisition, we gradually try to shift to a hands-off manner. In addition, considering the importance of the movement of both hands in ADL, we maintain a basic attitude of conducting training without suppressing the movements of the upper limb on the nonparalyzed side. We specifically focus on the following nine points:

(i) Daily routine movements should be adequately included in the training tasks.
(ii) All factors of gross motor, dexterity, and combined movements (by both hands) should be included in the training tasks.
(iii) The upper limb portion to be focused on during training should be clearly shown.
(iv) The functional training should be conducted in a step-by-step manner toward the acquisition of movements and activities.
(v) A lot of movements which the patient can continue in self-exercise at home or in the ADL after discharge should be included in the training.
(vi) In principle, the upper limb on the nonparalyzed side should not be restrained.
(vii) Feedback about the movements should be delivered not only by verbal instructions but also by manual intervention.
(viii) The patient's images of the movements and activities should be enhanced by describing the training contents in detail every time and obtaining his/her understanding, Immediately after admission to the hospital, gross motor exercise accounts for the majority of the training, approximately 80 %. The training program should be structured so that the dexterity motion and combined motion exercise will increase over time and finally account for the majority of the program.
(ix) The patient's active attitude and our assistance in his/her training and learning should be emphasized during the training. It is important to show our support for the patient by giving positive feedback.

a. Training Structure

Our training structure can be roughly classified into (i) gross motor movement, (ii) functional training including dexterity motions, and (iii) applied training including combined motions. During hospitalization, the proportions of these three types of training are gradually changed depending on the stage, as shown in Fig. 2.3.

Patients with poststroke hemiparesis have specific motion patterns such as hypotonic in the central portion (proximal muscle), unnatural hypertonic in the peripheral portion (distal muscle), and labored motions especially when starting up. Given these facts, patients should start mainly with gross motor training focusing on facilitations to improve the bearing properties of the central portion and to reduce hypertension in the peripheral portion. Subsequently, we try to gradually increase the percentage of facilitation training of the distal portions while improving the bearing properties of the central portion.

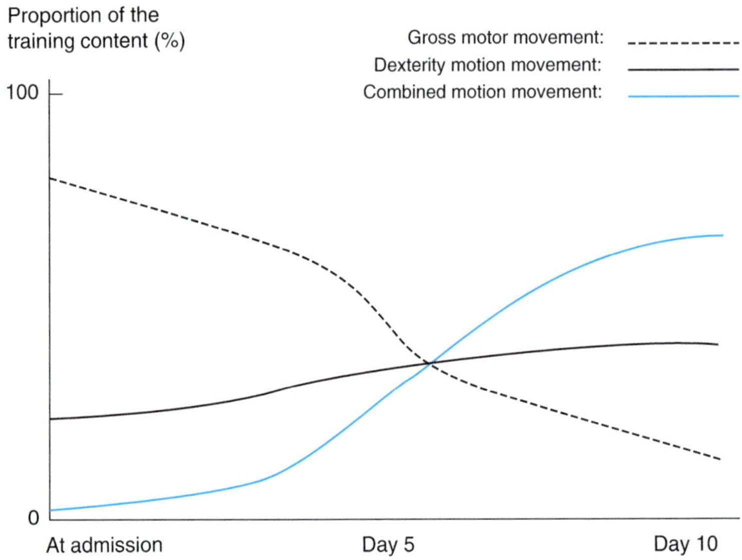

Fig. 2.3 Changes in weighting of the training content in NEURO-15
Immediately after admission to the hospital, gross motor exercise accounts for the majority of the training, approximately 80 %. The training program should be structured so that the dexterity motion and combined motion exercise will increase over time and finally account for the majority of the program

In practice, we make an intervention to improve the bearing properties and endurance of the body trunk and the center of the upper limb so that the function of the central portion, which is considered important in reaching movements, can be improved. In dexterity motion training, we conduct exercises such as facilitation to move the distal portion individually, as well as an object manipulation exercise to improve grasping and manipulating movements.

b. Points of the Combined Motion Training (by Both Hands)

In combined motion training, we conduct motion training directly linked to the actual ADL, focusing on bimanual actions based on the patient's needs in a step-by-step manner. ADL movements in particular require coordinated motions of both hands. As described above, however, many patients receive different sensory information from the upper limb on the paralyzed side compared to before their stroke and show poor bimanual movements and activities by learned nonuse.

Therefore, in the one-to-one OT, we provide guidance and intervention to reacquire the coordination of both hands such as in eating and grooming. In life during hospitalization as well, we instruct patients to actively use the upper limb on the paralyzed side and to repeatedly learn how to do motions and activities. In combined motion training, we consider to use self-help equipment in some cases and develop ideas to achieve the patient's needs and goals as much as possible.

Combined motion training is introduced around the midterm of hospitalization. However, in some cases, such as patients who are good at isolated movement and simply have a problem of learned nonuse, we proactively introduce bimanual motion training and ADL and IADL training from the start-up period and make a flexible intervention according to the severity of motor paresis and usage of the paralyzed side.

In this way, patients undertake functional training and relearn how to move in NEURO-15. They tend to get a "good response" compared to before admission, with comments such as "Now I can move more easily," "My movements are getting smoother," and "There are more things I can do." As a result, the patient's mind and attitude about the upper limb on the paralyzed side changes, and he/she starts thinking that he/she "tries to" or "wants to" use it in the ADL. We believe that habitual repetitive practice can help improve the frequency of use of the upper limb on the paralyzed side and effectively eliminate the learned nonuse.

3) Self-Exercise Program

An inpatient does a self-exercise program by himself/herself based on the prepared handouts that indicate the points of the self-exercise and cautions to review the training in one-to-one OT. If a problem occurs in the self-exercise, it should be reviewed in the next one-to-one OT with help from the therapist in charge. We create a self-exercise program after discharge including important points about the acquired movements in the self-exercise during hospitalization. Our handouts show ADL settings where the patient can use the upper limb on the paralyzed side. Thus, we have developed ideas to give the patient a specific image of using the upper limb on the paralyzed side in ADL. In addition, we provide an explanation about improved functions, acquired movements, and how to do the self-exercise also to supportive family members at the time of discharge, which can help them understand the current status of the patient's dysfunction and recovery.

4) Actual Training Program

a. Gross Motor Training

Movement patterns specific to chronic stroke patients include central hypotonia and peripheral unnatural hypertonia. Therefore, at the start of one-to-one OT, we make an intervention focusing on the gross motor training shown in Fig. 2.4 in order to improve voluntary properties, bearing properties, and endurance of the central portion and to reduce tension in the peripheral portion.

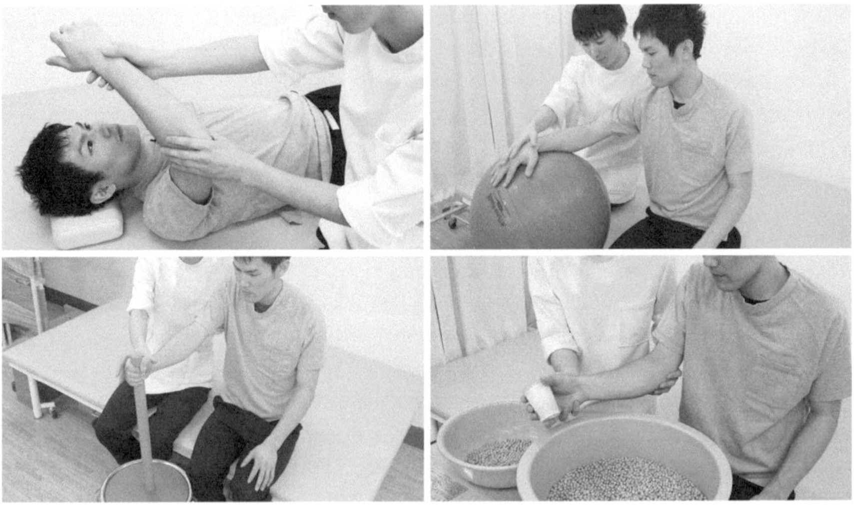

Fig. 2.4 Gross motor training

b. Dexterity Motion Training

Dexterity motion training is introduced at the same time as the gross motor training, and we make an intervention to gradually increase the percentage of facilitation training in the peripheral portion. Typical types of training are shown in Fig. 2.5.

c. Combined Motion Training

Combined motion training including bimanual behaviors, such as object manipulation training and ADL, is applied when the patient has already acquired the voluntary wrist's movement to some extent, when the patient can gradually move the wrist joint individually, or around the midterm of the training intervention. Typical training types are shown in Fig. 2.6.

3 Treatment Results of the Multicenter Trial: Introduction of Multicenter Data

In April 2008, our group started NEURO, which is a combination treatment of low-frequency rTMS and the intensive OT for poststroke patients with upper limb hemiparesis. As mentioned above, after confirming its efficacy and safety in a few cases, we have extensively conducted its 15-day protocol called NEURO-15 since April 2009.

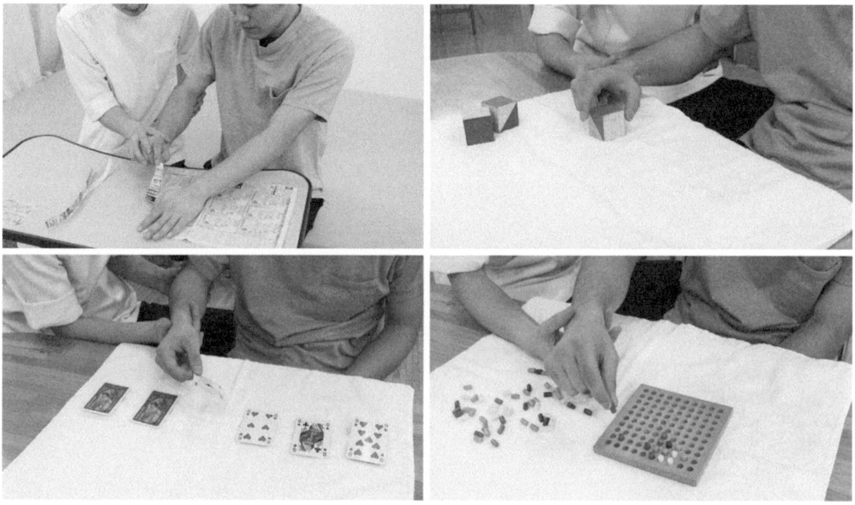

Fig. 2.5 Dexterity movement training

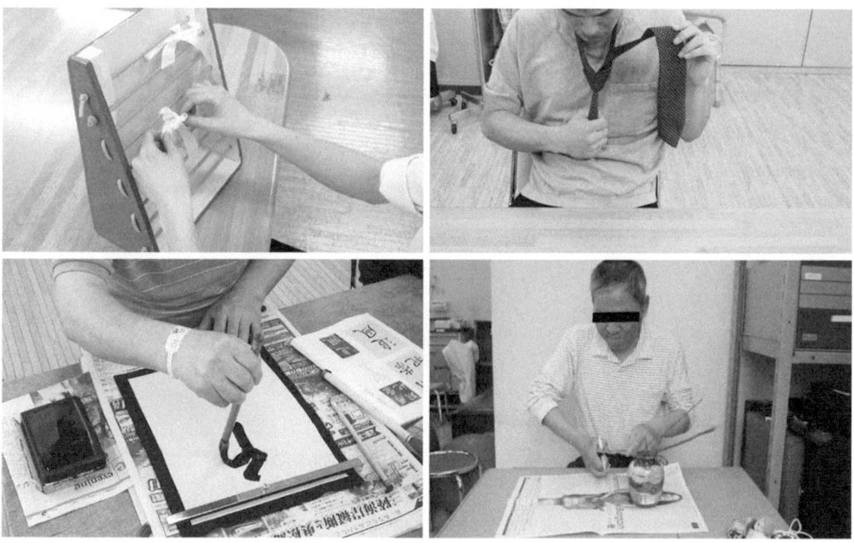

Fig. 2.6 Combined motion training

The protocol is now being conducted in the 11 institutions shown in Fig. 2.7. As of October 31, 2014, the protocol had been applied to a total of 2008 patients in 13 institutions (2 institutions are not currently providing the protocol for some reason). In this section, however, we show the data as of August 31, 2012, when the protocol had been applied to a total of 1008 patients. This data was published in *Japanese*

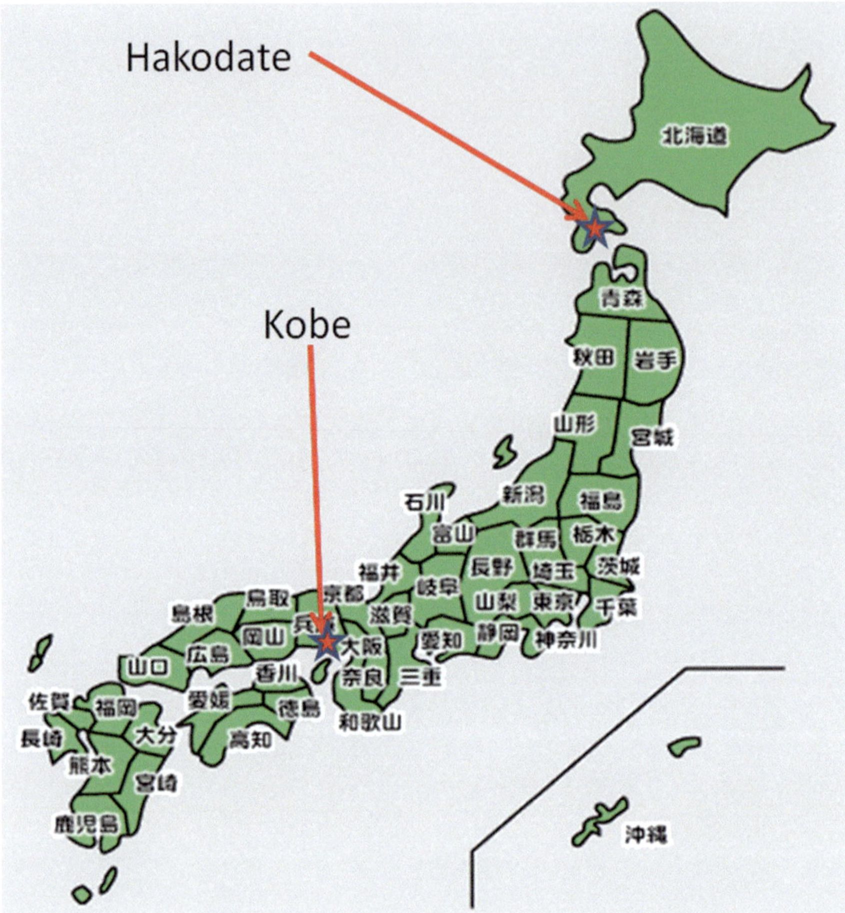

Fig. 2.7 List of the institutions conducting NEURO-15 (As of November 1, 2014)

Journal of Stroke in 2013 [20]. At that time, the protocol was being conducted in eight institutions.

The eight institutions include the following:

The Jikei University Hospital (Minato-Ku, Tokyo)
The Jikei University Daisan Hospital (Komae, Tokyo)
Shimizu Hospital, The Kyosaikai Medical Foundation (Kurayoshi, Tottori)
Tokyo General Hospital, The Kenkoukai Medical Foundation (Nakano, Tokyo)
Nishi-Hiroshima Rehabilitation Hospital, The Houwakai Medical Corporation (Hiroshima, Hiroshima)
Kimura Hospital, The Jujinkai Medical Corporation (Sabae, Fukui)
Aizawa Hospital, The Jisenkai Social Welfare Juridical Person (Matsumoto, Nagano)

Suwa no Mori Hospital, The Koshinkai Medical Corporation (Oita, Oita)
For some reasons, Aizawa Hospital and Suwa no Mori Hospital ended the provision of the protocol before November, 2014.

A. Overview of the Study Patients

The report on this multicenter study includes 1008 patients who visited 1 of the 8 institutions during the period of April 1, 2009, to August 31, 2012, and wanted to participate in NEURO-15 and met all the eligibility criteria described above.

The clinical backgrounds of the study patients are shown in Table 2.12 [20]. The mean age at admission was 61.1 ± 12.4 years, and the mean elapsed time from stroke onset to treatment was 81.5 ± 88.5 months. With regard to the subtypes of stroke, 522 patients with intracerebral hemorrhage and 486 patients with cerebral infarction were included. While 570 patients had dominant upper limb hemiparesis, 438 patients had nondominant upper limb hemiparesis.

B. Training Contents

The training content of NEURO-15 was as follows:

(i) Low-frequency rTMS was performed for the patient in sitting position using MagPro R30 and a figure-8 coil.
(ii) Stimulation was performed on the site where the largest MEP in the FDI muscle of the upper limb on the nonparalyzed side can be elicited within the primary motor area of the nonlesional hemisphere.
(iii) The intensity was set at 90 % of the motor threshold of the muscle (the minimum stimulus intensity that can produce MEP at the stimulation site).

Table 2.12 Clinical characteristics of patients treated with NEURO-15

Age at the intervention, years [range]		61.1 ± 12.4 [18–90]
Gender	Female	337 (33 %)
	Male	671 (67 %)
Time after stroke onset, months		81.5 ± 88.5 [12–338]
Subtype of stroke	Intracerebral hemorrhage	522 (52 %)
	Cerebral infarction	486 (48 %)
Side of upper limb hemiparesis	Dominant hand	570 (57 %)
	Non-dominant hand	438 (43 %)
Brunnstrom Recovery Stage for hand-fingers	Stage 3	202 (20 %)
	Stage 4	360 (36 %)
	Stage 4	446 (44 %)

Adopted from Ref. [20]

(iv) rTMS was immediately discontinued when an adverse event or adverse reaction occurred.
(v) The protocol during hospitalization consisted of low-frequency rTMS and an intensive OT. One session of low-frequency rTMS of 1 Hz lasted 20 minutes (a total of 1200 pulses).
(vi) 120-minute intensive OT as a combination therapy consisted of 60-minute one-to-one OT and 60-minute self-exercise. Two sessions were performed every day except the day of admission, the day of discharge, and Sundays.
(vii) Upper limb motor function was evaluated by using FMA items related upper limb and WMFT log performance time.
(viii) Upper limb function was evaluated at admission, at discharge, and at 4 weeks after discharge.

C. Training Results

First, we describe the safety of the protocol. All 204 patients completed NEURO-15, and no one showed a change in vital signs, such as blood pressure and pulse. Exacerbation of neurological findings and deterioration of motor function were not observed in any patient. Of the 1008 patients who completed this protocol, 271 patients were evaluated at 4 weeks after discharge. Of these 271 patients, none showed any adverse reactions during the 4 weeks after discharge.

Viewing the evaluations of 204 patients at admission and discharge, FMA showed a significant improvement from 45.3 ± 12.1 points to 49.7 ± 10.4 points (Fig. 2.8) [20], while WMFT log performance time also improved significantly from 2.78 ± 1.07 to 2.43 ± 1.22 (Fig. 2.9) [20].

The FMA score of the 271 patients who were evaluated at 4 weeks after discharge was 46.7 ± 10.5 points, 50.6 ± 8.7 points, and 49.9 ± 9.3 points at admission, at discharge, and at 4 weeks after discharge, respectively. These results indicate that both the scores at discharge and at 4 weeks after discharge showed a significant improvement compared to that at admission (Fig. 2.10) [20].

WMFT log performance time shifted from 2.46 ± 1.30, 2.11 ± 1.29, to 2.18 ± 1.37. It also showed a significant improvement at discharge and at 4 weeks after discharge compared to that at admission (Fig. 2.11) [20].

Both the log performance time of FMA and WMFT showed a significant improvement at 4 weeks after discharge as well, which indicates that the improvement of the motor function can be maintained even at 4 weeks after receiving NEURO-15.

The multicenter study described above demonstrated that the current protocol of NEURO-15 is safe and highly effective as well as generally feasible in many institutions.

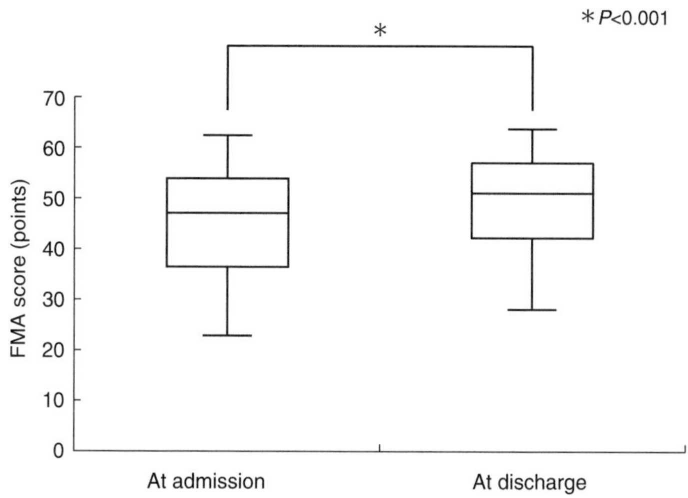

Fig. 2.8 Change in FMA score in patients receiving NEURO-15. FMA score at discharge showed a significant improvement compared to that at admission [20]

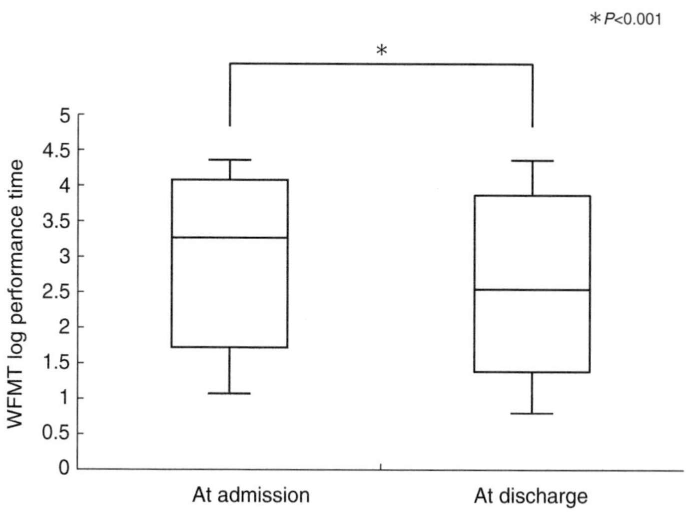

Fig. 2.9 Change in WFMT log performance time in patients receiving NEURO-15. WFMT log performance time showed a significant improvement compared to that at admission [20]

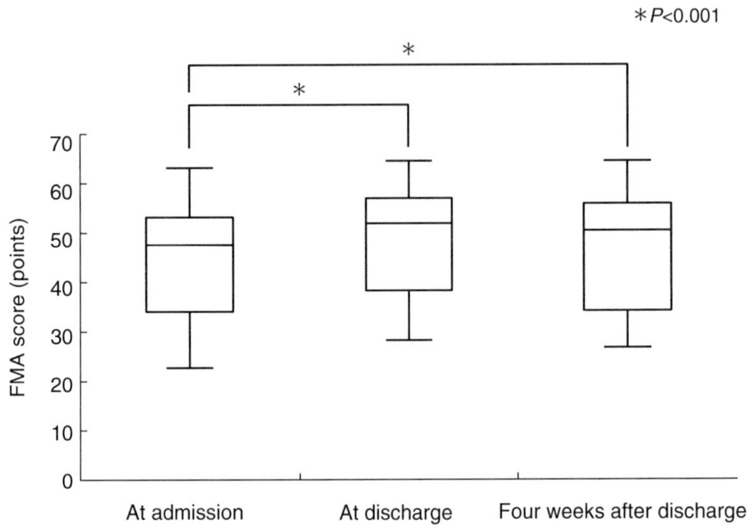

Fig. 2.10 Evaluation at four weeks after discharge and change in FMA score in evaluated patients. FMA score at discharge and at four weeks after discharge showed a significant improvement compared to that at admission [20]

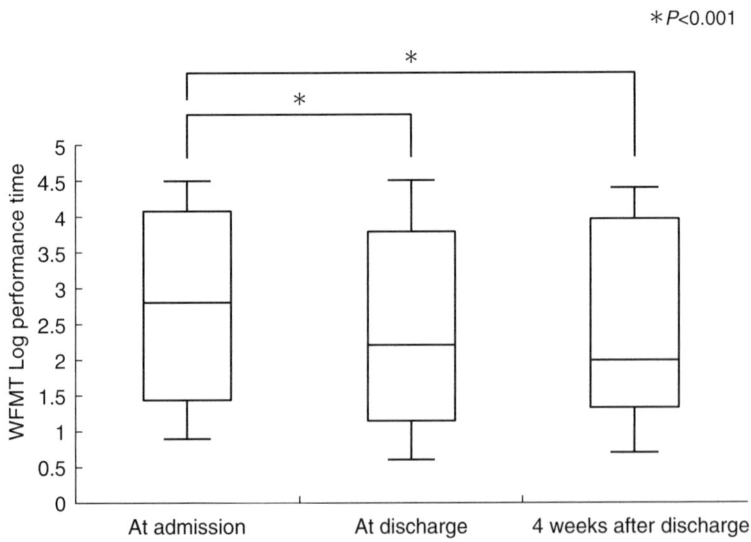

Fig. 2.11 Evaluation at four weeks after discharge and change in WFMT log performance time in evaluated patients. WFMT log performance time at discharge and at four weeks after discharge showed a significant improvement compared to that at admission [20]

4 Efforts by Each Institution for Improving the Quality of rTMS Treatment

As described above, the safety and efficacy of NEURO-15 has been demonstrated with the results of the previous studies. From past experience, we consider that OT is essential in NEURO-15 and there is a possibility that OT may contribute to improving poststroke upper limb hemiparesis by producing synergies with rTMS, which eliminates the imbalance of interhemispheric inhibition. While NEURO-15 is currently being conducted at 11 institutions, each institution is still learning through trial and error and seeking more effective interventions through consideration and generating unique ideas. Efforts by each institution are described as follows.

A. Combined Therapy with PT

In rTMS in NEURO-15, stimulation is performed to the primary motor area of the nonlesional hemisphere, where the largest MEP in the FDI muscle of the unaffected upper limb can be elicited.

In Penfield's homunculus (p. 104), the area responsible for the lower limb function is located near the fissura interhemisphaerica at considerable depth. Thinking anatomically, it is difficult to have a positive effect on the lower limb motor function through magnetic stimulation with a figure-8 used in NEURO-15. However, 20–30 % of patients who received stimulation to the upper limb motor area actually felt an effect on lower limb motor function. This suggests the possibility that if the plasticity around the cerebral lesions responsible for upper limb functions has increased after stroke onset, not only the area near the fissura interhemisphaerica but also the area responsible for lower limb function can be recovered.

In addition, most patients who are hospitalized to receive NEURO-15 hope to improve their walking ability as well as upper limb motor function, and many ask us to perform combination therapy with physical therapy (PT). In general, many patients with stroke undertake self-exercise after discharge from a recovery phase rehabilitation hospital and continue rehabilitation with the use of long-term care. However, some patients are hospitalized to receive NEURO-15 1 year or more after stroke onset without receiving sufficient training or even without using an adequate brace.

Therefore, some institutions employ combination rehabilitation with PT to improve the lower limb motor function and walking function. In exercise therapy for improving the lower limb motor function, we make a therapeutic intervention with emphasis on facilitation exercise and stretch exercise of the muscle spasticity based on the degree of recovery of the lower limb on the paralyzed side as well as trunk muscle training through basic movements such as getting up and standing up. We also perform applied gait training, including balance training in a standing position and stair-climbing, to improve practical lower limb ability.

According to a recent report, a significant improvement in both walking and balance ability was observed in patients receiving CI therapy after performing combined treatment with PT focusing on walking compared to the preintervention period [21]. Intensive rehabilitation during hospitalization similar to CI therapy is also being performed in our ongoing NEURO-15. We believe that this is useful and highly satisfactory for patients who can "re-learn" by therapeutic rehabilitative intervention.

B. Training Using Photos or Videos

As needed, many institutions give patients feedback using photos and videos. Mancebo et al. [22] and van Vliet et al. [23] reported that visual feedback using photos and videos is useful in rehabilitation for poststroke upper limb hemiparesis unless the patient has visual impairment, unilateral spatial neglect, or severe impaired attention. We consider that these kinds of visual feedback help patients understand a specific posture and motion images and can also improve the patient's motivation during the training period.

Many institutions utilize these types of training in self-exercise and guidance after discharge, described below. They take photos of activities in daily life which the patient could successfully achieve during hospitalization and prepare unique manuals along with easy-to-understand advice. At discharge, these institutions give the patient these materials along with a self-exercise program and provide guidance to keep using the upper limb on the paralyzed side at home.

C. Devices About Self-Exercise Program

Each institution has come up with its own approach to self-exercise program. The main goal of self-exercise is to improve muscle strength and endurance, to perform motion repetition training, and to conduct task-oriented training to improve ADL. In this context, many institutions prepare achievable self-exercise programs tailored to the individual patient, which consist of not only basic training programs but also applied training related to cooking procedures and the patient's hobbies which were known through an interview at admission (Tables 2.13 and 2.14). These institutions conduct an occasional review of the self-exercise programs and intensity according to the patient's level of achievement and give feedback. The concept of a transfer package described below is also incorporated and utilized when creating self-exercise program.

Table 2.13 An example of a self-exercise program (1)[a]

Self-exercise program for Mr./Ms. XX XX
1. Ball lifting (20 times × 2 sets)
2. Wall wiping (up-and-down, 20 times × 2 sets) *If there is pain, please do this exercise moderately *Keep the right arm close to the body with the left hand on the wall to support yourself
3. Small pegs (peg and unpeg/invert) *Do this exercise while holding the peg with the ring and little fingers
4. Marble rolling (10 times per set) *Use large marbles *Roll them inside the palm of your hand
5. Applied training 1. Use chopsticks well 2. Write words well

[a]Take a rest when you feel tired

Table 2.14 An example of self- exercise program (2)[a]

Self-exercise program for Mr./Ms. XX XX
1. Lift a ball above your head with both hands (15 times × 2 sets)
2. Lift a ball at a right angle with both hands (15 times × 2 sets)
3. Spin a ball with both hands (15 times × 2 sets)
4. Do push-ups on a table (15 times)
5. Do push-ups against a wall
6. Stretch the medial rotator (maintain 10 seconds × 10 times)
7. Move thick pegs
8. Writing exercise

[a]Take a rest when you feel tired

Do not use my weaker arm at all (do not want to use it)

D. Evaluation and Direction After Discharge

Nakama [24] mentioned that self-exercise at home is not just voluntary training but behavioral modification from the patient and his/her family's dependent and passive activities to their proactive and positive activities. At the time of discharge from hospitalization for NEURO-15, the therapist explains the achievements and results during hospitalization and provides direction about self-exercise after discharge. Important points in self-exercise are first, to have the patient acquire the habit of "keeping on using the upper limb on the paralyzed side" in daily life after discharge; second, to maintain the acquired function, continue to provide guidance by assessing whether the patient is training correctly and making modifications when necessary; and finally, share the information not only with the patient and medical professionals but also with the patient's family.

Table 2.15 Directions of self-exercise

Evaluation	Body functions, activities, social environment, personality, and needs
Problem analysis	Share the problem and analyze what movements the patient needs. Make clear the purpose of the exercise
Goal setting	Set an achievable, sustainable and reasonable goal. Set a goal that offers an image of future life and a goal that should be achieved in the immediate future in accordance with the patient and his/her family's chief complaints and requests, as well as a prognosis based on an objective evaluation and problem analysis from the perspective of each medical profession
Exercise content setting	Exercise can include a movement that fits to the patient's body function, repetitive practice of living activities, or social participation itself. Create a specific exercise content
Monitoring	Check the patient's status when he/she visits the hospital or by phone. Ask him/her to shoot a video of his/her daily life and give feedback by reviewing it

Reference [24]

Nakama also said in the guidance for self-exercise after discharge that evaluation, problem analysis, goal setting, exercise content setting, and monitoring are important in intervention in self-exercise after discharge (Table 2.15) [24].

Based on these facts, each institution has tried to develop a variety of ideas. Many institutions encourage their patients to use movements acquired during hospitalization even in daily life after discharge and set a specific and achievable goal. Then, step-by-step exercises according to individual ability are shown in detail using illustrations and photos. In addition, as described above, patients are provided with training advice and photos taken during hospitalization which show the movements they successfully did or they became able to do through the exercise (Figs. 2.12 and 2.13).

One institution uses a mountain climbing analogy to encourage patients to understand the current status of the upper limb on the paralyzed side and what is needed in future exercise (Fig. 2.14). They also ask patients to record what has changed in daily life and try to support their behavior modification (Fig. 2.15). They use this record to understand the patient's situation in daily life after discharge and to provide guidance after discharge. Some institutions have onsite facilities for visiting rehabilitation or ambulatory rehabilitation, which enables them to provide continuous guidance even after discharge.

At the time of discharge, these institutions also provide an explanation and guidance about achievable movements to the family members to share information. Some institutions ask not only the patient but his/her family to check how the patient uses the upper limb on the paralyzed side at home and whether he/she is able to continue the exercise. In addition, they conduct an interview at four weeks after discharge to track activities of daily living and the exercise, which is reflected in the evaluation and future exercises, and again, some advice is provided by the medical staff.

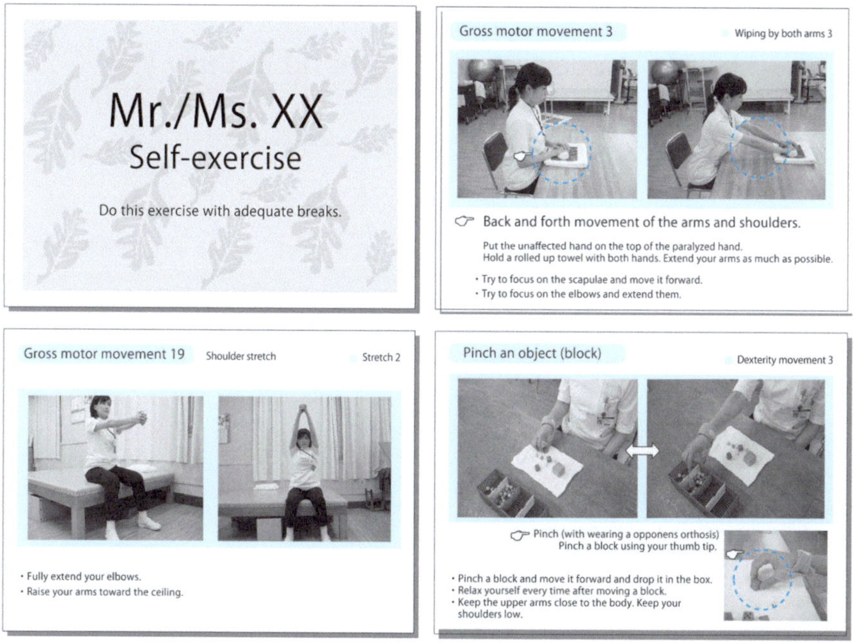

Fig. 2.12 An example of a booklet for guidance at the time of discharge (Jikei University Hospital)

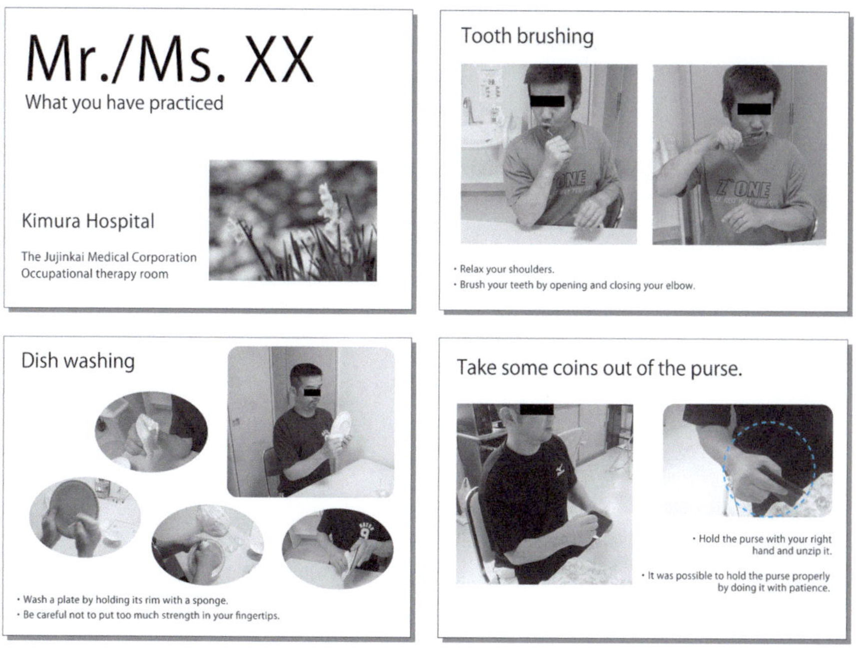

Fig. 2.13 An example of a booklet prepared for guidance at discharge (Kimura Hospital)

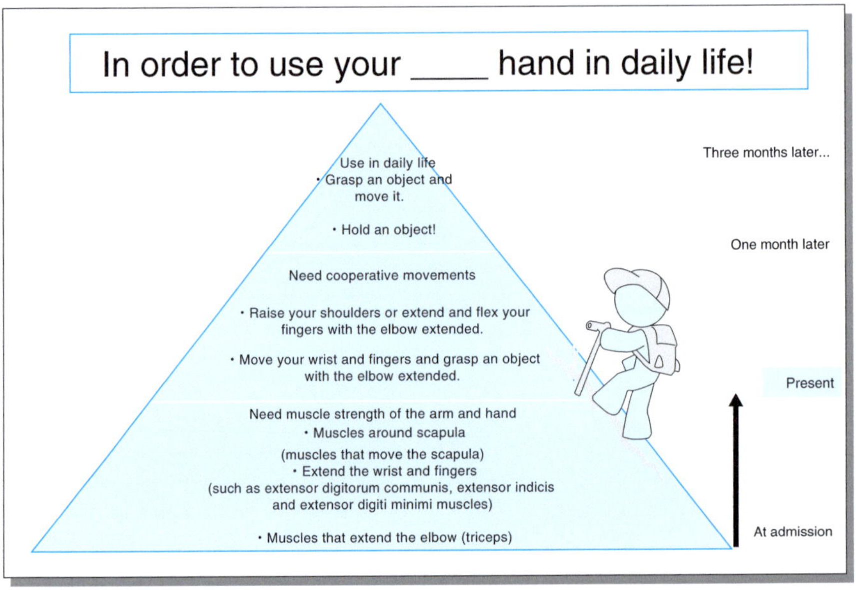

Fig. 2.14 Guidance to modify behaviors at and after discharge. This institution gives an explanation using easy-to-understand illustrations so that the patient can understand the status of his/her paresis at discharge and make an effort to improve the motivation and modify behaviors (Data provided by Aizawa Hospital)

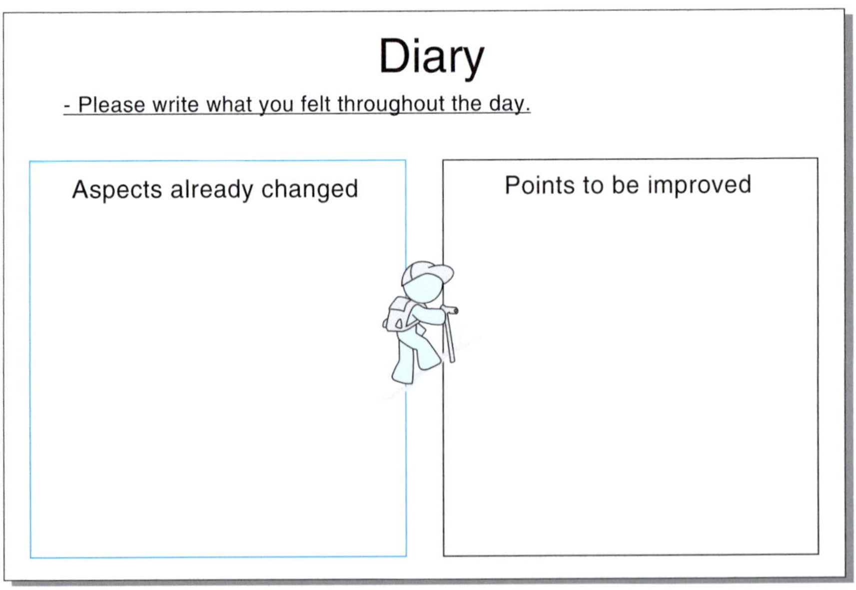

Fig. 2.15 Record-keeping form for patients to facilitate behavior modification after discharge (Data provided by Aizawa Hospital)

E. Initiatives During Hospital Ward Life

As a rule, a hospitalization for NERUO-15 lasts 15 days. To efficiently promote behavioral modification and improvement of the upper limb on the paralyzed side during this short period, nurses at some institutions check how patients use the upper limb on the paralyzed side during their stay in the hospital ward. It is important that nurses understand the patient's use of the upper limb on the paralyzed side, something that might be difficult for physicians and therapists, and identify the patient's problems and concerns about the use of the upper limb on the paralyzed side through communication with the patient. One institution uses its own checklist shown in Fig. 2.16 and encourages patients to use the upper limb on the paralyzed side during their time in the hospital ward, including use in the early morning and at night.

F. Application of the Transfer Package

The transfer package is a strategy of efficient occupational therapy in CIMT proposed by Taub et al. [25] and Morris et al. [26] in 2006. It is a behavioral strategy to increase the frequency of use of the hand on the paralyzed side and improve the quality of movement in the ADL in real life. Many patients have not only a dysfunction caused by post-stroke upper limb hemiparesis but also a behavioral disorder due to the nonuse of the upper limb on the paralyzed side. Therefore, with the transfer package shown in Table 2.16, the therapist and the patient plan a behavioral strategy to improve the upper limb on the paralyzed side during hospitalization and conduct training to overcome barriers and to sustain its effect even after discharge. A major difference between the transfer package and the traditional training is that in the latter, a patient is passively provided with his/her exercise contents and training methods by a therapist and that in the former patient and therapist cooperate to create training methods and steps to achieve the next goal. This will be described in detail along with the contents of Table 2.16.

(i) In monitoring, use the MAL at the time of admission as a subjective evaluation measure to understand the status of the ADL and assess how the patient uses the upper limb on the paralyzed side in self-exercise and in ADL and how the training is proceeding.
(ii) In problem solving, pick out hard-to-do movements in daily life and during hospitalization, consider why they are hard to do, and have the patient work on a solution to make them possible.
(iii) In behavioral contract, clarify the role of the upper limb on the paralyzed side in daily life and during hospitalization, and make it clear (promise) that the patient should work on the selected solution and use the upper limb on the paralyzed side in daily life.

Rating scale of the use of the paralyzed side in daily life

Name ( ) Age (years old) Male / Female Dominant hand (right / left) Paralyzed side (right / left)							
Rating 0: cannot do 1: can do 2: can do with a self-help tool or environmental adjustment 3: always do							
Evaluated movement		Day 3	Day 5	Day 7	Day 9	Day 11	Day 13
		Mon	Wed	Fri	Sun	Tue	Thu
Eating	Can eat with both hands.						
	Can use chopsticks or a spoon with the hand on the paralyzed side.						
	Can hold a plate or keep it from moving with the hand on the paralyzed side.						
Grooming	Can wash your hands with both hands.						
Dressing	Can put on a shirt and take it off using both hands.						
Daily activities	Can take out a piece of tissue paper with the hand on the paralyzed side.						
	Can take a bill out of your wallet with the hand on the paralyzed side.						
	Can take a coin out of your purse with the hand on the paralyzed side.						
Physical status	Can move the thumb on the paralyzed side and touch all the other fingertips in order from the index finger. (1: index finger, 2: middle finger, 3: ring finger, 4: little finger)						
	Can raise the hand on the paralyzed side. (0: 45° or less, 1: 90°, 2: 135°, 3: 180°)						
Targeted movement							
Others							
Catch up test (Put an object on the table)							
Ball							
Pencil (Put it in parallel with your body)							
Paper (Can grasp the top of creaseless paper)							
Total score							

[Data provided by Suwa No Mori Hospital]

Fig. 2.16 Checklist of use of the upper limb on the paralyzed side in the hospital ward (Data provided by Suwa No Mori Hospital)

Table 2.16 What is the transfer package?

1. Monitoring	Monitoring of the training status and the use of the upper limb on the paralyzed side
2. Problem solving	Strategic planning of how to solve the problem in practice
3. Behavioral contract	Promise to work on solving the problem and to use the upper limb on the paralyzed side in daily life
4. Home skill assignment	List of activities conducted regularly
5. Home practice	Self-exercise at home
6. Daily schedule	Record of daily activities

(iv) In home skill assignment, gather information about the status of movements in daily life through an interview, evaluate the patient's needs and the result of the MAL, and reflect the feedback in the exercise.

(v) After that, conduct self-exercise (home practice) every day in addition to the training provided by the therapist, and continue updating suitable self-exercises for the individual patient on a daily basis.

(vi) As a daily schedule, record the activities and training details in daily life, have the patient understand the contents and review them, and make it possible to provide feedback about the qualitative changes of the upper limb on the paralyzed side.

Currently, some institutions are attempting to introduce this transfer package. A difference between the transfer package and the traditional exercises in NEURO-15 is that a patient is not passively provided with training and self-exercise plans created by a therapist, but rather the patient sets goals to promote behavioral modifications and voluntarily works on the exercises. However, the introduction of this transfer package in NEURO-15 has some problems: first, the status of the upper limb on the paralyzed side and the background of life differ from one patient to another; second, not all patients can always act on their own initiative. We think that there is room for further consideration.

G. Introduction of COPM

Each institution has developed its own ideas as described above. Under these circumstances, it is important to enable the patient to receive the maximum effect within a short period of time and to direct him/her to keep on doing the exercise after discharge. When the evaluation is made at the time of admission, it is sometimes difficult to set goals because some patients do not clearly understand the status of the upper limb on the paralyzed side and their own needs in ADL. In other words, there are occasionally cases that cannot be addressed by bottom-up rehabilitation. Therefore, one institution has attempted to introduce the Canadian occupational performance measure (COPM) to solve this problem.

COPM is an individual measure developed by Law et al. [27] and was created to evaluate a patient's perception over time when performing an occupation. In the occupational performance model in COPM, it is considered that an occupation is performed as a result of the interaction between a person, an occupation, and the environment. The occupations comprise three categories, namely, self-care, productive activities, and leisure: self-care means occupations by which patients keep themselves in good condition in daily life; productive activities include economic activities, daily housework, and school activities; leisure includes recreation other than their jobs or responsibilities.

We believe that a balance among these three categories is essential to perform an occupation and how well a therapist brings out the patient's skills as a performance element is important. This means that it is a top-down method provided at the first visit to bring out the performance element and utilize it in the exercise. A patient who is considered at the first visit to be unable to obtain a sufficient effect from the bottom-up method only requires intensive rehabilitation, including the top-down method. We think this should be reviewed in future studies.

5 Effect of rTMS on Spasticity

Through rehabilitation for patients with stroke in daily clinical practice, we have realized that many patients have spasticity along with hemiplegia.

Spasticity is observed in various ways. In some cases, it occurs when moving and inhibits the movement. In contrast, other patients conduct movement by using the spasticity. In the recovery process of poststroke patients with hemiparesis, muscle tonus and increased reflex are necessary to some extent. If spasticity occurs, however, the patient suffers from an awkwardness of movement and a pain as well as an impairment of ADL and the quality of life (QOL) [28]. Although we try to develop rehabilitation to enable patients to actively control muscle tonus, it is actually very difficult to achieve.

In recent years, an increasing number of studies have reported that better therapeutic effects have been obtained by performing rehabilitation after using medication or physical devices to reduce the excessively increased spasticity. The clinical application of rTMS by our group seems to be one of these studies [29]. In this section, we will describe the pathophysiology and the evaluation method of spasticity as well as the effect of rTMS on spasticity.

A. Pathophysiology of Spasticity

According to reports from Western countries, the frequency of spasticity occurrence in stroke patients increases with the time course of the disease: the incidence at 3 months and at 12 months after stroke is approximately 19 % and 38 %, respectively [30, 31].

The most well-known definition of spasticity proposed by Lance [32] in 1980 is that "Spasticity is a motor disorder characterized by a velocity-dependent increase in tonic stretch reflexes (muscle tone) with exaggerated tendon jerks, resulting from hyper-excitability of the stretch reflex, as one component of the upper motor neuron syndrome."

The diseases that cause upper motor neuron disorders include cerebrovascular disorder, cerebral palsy, head trauma, spinal cord injury, and multiple sclerosis. The neurological symptoms are classified into positive and negative symptoms. The positive symptoms include spasticity (findings such as increased muscle tone, exaggerated tendon jerks, stretch reflexes that affect other muscles and clonus) as well as focal dystonia, pathological synergy, pathological cocontraction, and increased flexor reflex such as Babinski reflex. The negative symptoms include a decrease in muscle output, muscle weakness including bradykinesia, motor paralysis, impaired isolated movement, dexterity impairment, easy fatigability, and impaired selective activities of the individual muscle.

Upper motor neurons act as neuronal pathways from the motor area of the cerebral cortex to neuronal cell bodies located in the anterior horn of the spinal cord at various levels. When part of them develop impairment such as mechanical damage, vascular insufficiency, and degeneration, an inhibitory signal to the reflex center located in the lower part of the brainstem and the spinal cord is reduced and is freed from control. It is thought that the excessive muscle tone and the increased spinal reflexes occur and the excitability of the spinal motor cells increase, which cause spasticity.

However, there is an opinion that spasticity does not occur when the pyramidal tract (including medullary pyramidal tract and lateral corticospinal tract), which is a projection path from the primary motor cortex corresponding to the Brodmann's area 4 to the spinal cord, is selectively damaged, while it occurs when the pyramidal tract is damaged along with Brodmann's area 6 [33]. There is also another opinion that spasticity occurs by dysregulation of reticulospinal and vestibulospinal tract which are inhibitory descending tracts [34].

The alpha motor neurons that control extrafusal muscle fibers and the gamma motor neurons that control intrafusal muscle fibers are involved in the occurrence of spasticity. Spasticity is characterized by a pathological enhancement of phasic stretch reflexes, which is one of the skeletal muscle reflexes at the spinal level. The muscle spindle is stimulated when the muscle is passively stretched. This stimulus is transmitted to the spinal cord through group Ia neural fibers, which stimulates the alpha motor neurons of the muscle and causes the stretched muscle to contract reflexively (stretch reflex). Group Ia neural fibers also have inhibitory synaptic connections with alpha motor neurons which control the antagonist and cause its relaxation (reciprocal inhibition).

For this reason, it is considered that the upper motor neuron disorders cause increased muscle spindle sensitivity, reduced presynaptic inhibition at the terminal of group Ia fibers, sprouting and formation of group Ia fibers, increased sensitivity of postsynaptic membrane, increased excitatory input, or reduced inhibitory input to alpha motor neurons, which results in enhanced stretch reflexes and the impairment of reciprocal inhibition [35].

On the other hand, when gamma motor neurons are stimulated by impulses from the upper central nervous system, the intrafusal muscle fibers contract, and the activity of group Ia neural fibers are increased. This increase is transmitted to alpha motor neurons via the dorsal root, which promotes the stimulation. Such a pathway is called a gamma loop, and this reaction is also a mechanism that brings an increase in muscle tone. The descending tract from the upper central nervous system can indirectly control the activity of group Ia neural fibers in order to regulate the activity of gamma motor neurons. This means that the sustained activity of alpha motor neurons can also be controlled by the descending tract. When the activity of gamma motor neurons is increased, the muscle becomes more rigid and shows resistance to bending and stretching exercises. This is the increased muscle tone.

The combination of increased stretch reflexes and increased muscle tone caused through this process is considered spasticity. While the detailed pathophysiology of spasticity is still unclear, there is no objection that spasticity appears when descending information signals from the upper central nervous system to the spinal neural circuit become affected.

B. Evaluation of Spasticity

MAS and modified Tardieu scale (MTS) are the typical evaluation indices of spasticity. In particular, there have been many reports using MAS in Japan and overseas due to its simplicity.

MAS is an evaluation measure proposed by Bohannon et al. [36], who modified the Ashworth scale developed by Ashworth in 1964 and improved its accuracy. A patient's feeling of resistance when a joint is passively moved over the maximum ROM of each joint for 1 second (how much resistance he/she felt at what point in time) is recorded and evaluated. However, there are conflicting reports on MAS for poststroke patients with hemiparesis: some show that MAS has the interrater reliability, while others take the opposing view. When a detailed examination is required, the combined use with electrophysiological test is preferable. Typical examples of the electrophysiological test for spasticity include F-wave and H-wave.

1) Evaluation by F-Wave

When the peripheral nerve is electrically stimulated in a vigorous manner, the large wave that first appears on the monitor is called the M wave (the summation of muscle action potential), and the subsequent wave is called the F-wave. The F-wave is a compound action potential resulting from the innervated muscle by electrical stimulation. The F-wave is thought to appear as an excitatory stimulation transmitted through alpha motor neurons in a retrograde fashion and reignites after being transmitted to the anterior horn cells in the spinal cord, before being transmitted again through the same alpha motor neurons in an antegrade fashion, with the consequence that an F-wave is recorded [37].

The F-wave can be recorded in various muscles, but excitation of neurons occurs only approximately once every 10–100 times. For this reason, if a surface electrode is used for recording, the excitation of several motor units is recorded in a single stimulation, and its latent time, amplitude, and waveform vary every time [37]. With regard to the F-wave that estimates the nerve conduction velocity and the excitability of spinal motor neurons, Tsai et al. [38] reported that the amplitude of the F-wave in patients with neurological sequelae of stroke correlates with the severity of spasticity. In this context, it is currently recommended as a noninvasive, quantitative, and neurophysiological examination of spasticity.

In general, patients with spasticity show an increase in F-wave amplitude, the F/M ratio (the ratio of the maximum M-wave amplitude and the mean F-wave amplitude which were derived from the same muscle), and the frequency of F-wave appearance (the ratio of F-wave to total number of stimulations). In patients with spasticity, the F/M ratio increases to 5 % of the maximum amplitude or more, occasionally to 10 % of it. The frequency of appearance of 80 % or more suggests a presence of spasticity caused by upper motor neuron disorders.

2) Evaluation by H-Wave

The H-wave, which was named after its discoverer Hoffmann, is the potential corresponding to the deep tendon reflexes and is regarded as a simple method to record spinal reflexes. The group Ia neural fibers, or the afferent nerves in the stretch reflex, are excited by electrical stimulation in antegrade manner, which generates an impulse and makes synaptic connections in the spinal cord. The postsynaptic potential then excites the motor nerves in the anterior horn cells in spinal cord. When its potential reaches the innervated muscle through alpha motor neurons, the H-wave is recorded.

However, the afferent nerves include the group Ia neural fibers that originate from the Golgi tendon organ. It is difficult to excite only the group Ia neural fibers in the muscle; therefore, the same waveform does not always appear in each stimulation [39]. In healthy adults, the muscles where the H-wave can be detected are limited to the quadriceps, soleus muscle, and flexor carpi radialis. However, the H-wave can also be detected in certain other muscles when performing a weak voluntary contraction.

It is known that patients with spasticity show an increase in the H/M ratio (the ratio of the maximum M-wave amplitude and the maximum H-wave amplitude that were derived from the same muscle). While an association with the severity of spasticity and the H/M ratio has not been found, it is believed that it helps objectively evaluate the time course of the same patient.

C. Effect of rTMS on Spasticity

rTMS is expected to regulate the excitability by providing stimulus to the cerebral cortex and to promote the smooth transmission of information signals between the upper central nervous system and the spinal cord. rTMS includes low-frequency rTMS, which is performed on the primary motor area in the nonlesional hemisphere, and high-frequency rTMS, which is performed on the primary motor area in the affected hemisphere. Both are recognized for their antispasticity effect.

1) Reports on High-Frequency rTMS

Centonze et al. [40] performed high-frequency rTMS at 5 Hz for 15 minutes (1 cycle consisted of 10 seconds of 5 Hz stimulation and 40 seconds of rest, in a total of 18 cycles) in the lower limb area of the primary motor cortex in the affected hemisphere of multiple sclerosis patients with lower limb spasticity. This was performed for 2 weeks, and MAS and the H/M ratio of the lower limb with spasticity were measured before and after the treatment.

As a result, high-frequency rTMS of 5 Hz instantaneously reduced the H/M ratio, with the reduction maintained also after performing daily treatment for 2 weeks. In accordance with this, the reduction of MAS was also observed after providing daily stimulation for 2 weeks. It was also confirmed that the reduction of both the H/M ratio and MAS was maintained for at least 1 week after the end of 2-week protocol.

Wupuer et al. [41] performed a total of 1000 pulses of high-frequency rTMS at 10 Hz (1 cycle consisted of 5 seconds of 10-Hz stimulation and 25 seconds of rest, in a total of 20 cycles) in the hand and finger area of the primary motor cortex in the affected hemisphere of patients with spasticity and neurological sequelae of stroke. The change in the F-wave was recorded before and after the treatment. Prior to the stimulation, the F-wave amplitude and F/M ratio in patients with neurological sequelae of stroke were significantly increased compared to those in healthy subjects. After performing high-frequency rTMS, however, the F/M ratio was significantly reduced.

These two reports suggest that high-frequency rTMS on the affected hemisphere eventually suppresses the excitability of the spinal cord. Therefore, we consider that it can be a therapeutic intervention for poststroke patients with upper limb hemiparesis.

2) Reports on Low-Frequency rTMS

Mály and Dinya [42] performed low-frequency rTMS and examined its effects in patients with stroke who had survived about 10 years after onset and had no change in the motor function for more than 5 years.

First, they performed single TMS on both hemispheres and classified the patients into four groups (Group A to D) according to the level of elicited upper limb movements. In Group A, rTMS was performed on both hemispheres (movements were elicited in both upper limbs). In Group B, rTMS was performed on the nonlesional hemisphere (movements were not elicited in either upper limb). In Group C, rTMS was performed on the affected hemisphere (movements were elicited only in the upper limb on the nonparalyzed side); and in Group D, rTMS was performed on the nonlesional hemisphere (movements were elicited only in the upper limb on the nonparalyzed side) (Table 2.17). Low-frequency rTMS 1 Hz, a total of 100 pulses (twice daily) was carried out on each stimulation site continuously for a week.

A reduction in spasticity was observed in each group 1 week after the treatment, and consequently the improvement continued for at least 1 month. Based on this, Málly and Dinya concluded that low-frequency rTMS can improve paralyzed limbs even if a patient has already reached a plateau state.

3) Reports by Our Group

It has been reported that NEURO-15 conducted by our group also has an antispasticity effect. Kakuda et al. [29] conducted NEURO-15 in poststroke patients with upper limb hemiparesis who have spasticity and assessed the degree of their upper limb motor function and upper limb spasticity before and after treatment. As a result, FMA and WMFT showed improvement in the motor function of the upper limb on the paralyzed side after 15 days of low-frequency rTMS and intensive OT. The reduction in muscle tonus in the upper limb flexors on the paralyzed side was also confirmed by the reduction in MAS.

Much of the mechanism by which rTMS brings about an antispasticity effect still remains unknown; however, we speculate that neural activation of the affected hemisphere can partly contribute. This is based on the finding that both high-frequency rTMS on the affected hemisphere and low-frequency rTMS on the nonlesional hemisphere reportedly increase the neural activity of the affected hemisphere and have anticonvulsant effects [40–42]. We consider that the increase in neural activities of the motor cortex of the affected hemisphere resulted in the increase in descending inhibitory input through the corticospinal tract, which suppressed the excitability of gamma and alpha motor neurons and reduced the spasticity of peripheral muscle (Fig. 2.17).

Table 2.17 Consideration by Málly and Dinya

<table>
<tr><th>Classification</th><th>Induction of movement</th><th>Stimulation sites</th></tr>
<tr><td>Group A</td><td>Observed in both upper limbs</td><td>Both hemisphere</td></tr>
<tr><td>Group B</td><td>Not observed in either upper limb</td><td>Non-lesional hemisphere</td></tr>
<tr><td>Group C</td><td rowspan="2">Observed only in the upper limb on the non-paralyzed side</td><td>Affected hemisphere</td></tr>
<tr><td>Group D</td><td>Non-lesional hemisphere</td></tr>
</table>

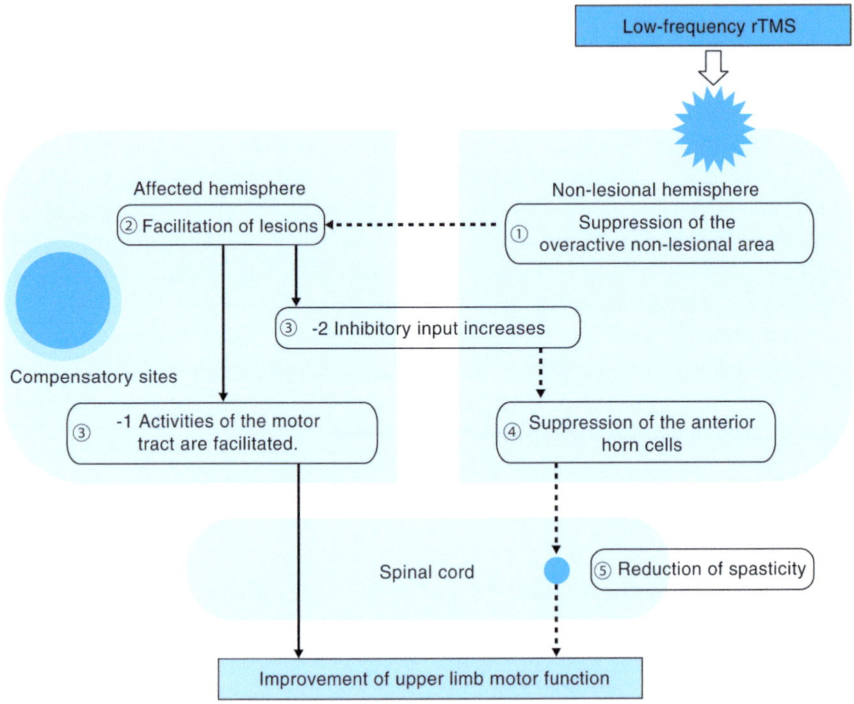

Fig. 2.17 Mechanism by which low-frequency rTMS brings about an anti-spasticity effect. Low-frequency rTMS on the non-lesional hemisphere increases the neural activity of the affected hemisphere, which promotes the activity of the motor system and results in a reduction of spasticity

Therefore, we conducted a study using the F-wave in poststroke patients to review the effects of low-frequency rTMS on the motor neuron excitability [43].

We examined 13 poststroke patients with upper limb hemiparesis who met all of our group's eligibility criteria of rTMS treatment (age: 57.5 ± 11.1 years old, elapsed time after onset: 55.2 ± 51.4 months, cerebral infarction: five patients, intracerebral hemorrhage: eight patients), after exclusion of those who received local injection of antispasticity drugs such as Botulinum Toxin Type A (BoNT-A).

The severity of the upper limb hemiparesis was assessed by using BRS for hand-fingers as a baseline. Among the study patients, seven patients were at stage IV, three patients were at stage V, and the other three patients were at state VI. The mean score of MAS was 0.62 ± 0.62 in the finger flexors and 0.73 ± 0.63 in the wrist flexors. Low-frequency rTMS at 1 Hz was applied on the hand finger area of the primary motor area in the nonlesional hemisphere of the study patients for 20 minutes. Before and after the treatment, the frequency of F-wave appearance and the F/M ratio were measured.

The results showed that, prior to the application of rTMS, the F/M ratio was significantly higher in the upper limb on the paralyzed side compared to that in the

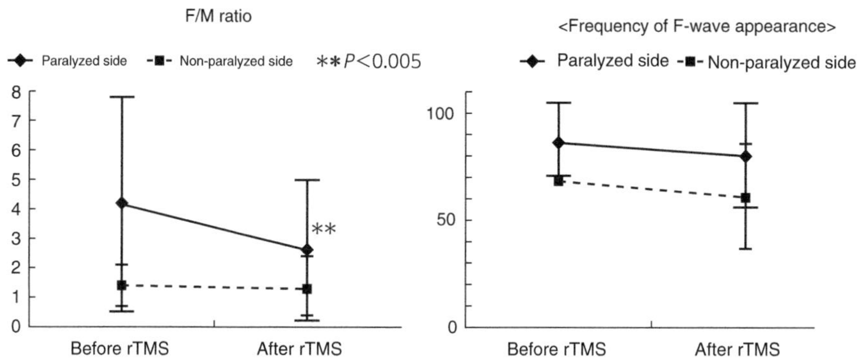

Fig. 2.18 Changes in the F/M ratio and the frequency of F-wave appearance by performing low-frequency rTMS. The F/M ratio of the upper limb on the paralyzed side was significantly reduced by low-frequency rTMS on the non-lesional hemisphere for 20 minutes [43]

upper limb on the nonparalyzed side. Low-frequency rTMS produced a downward trend in the frequency of F-wave appearance in the upper limbs both on the paralyzed and nonparalyzed side; however, its change was not statistically significant. A significant decrease in the F/M ratio was observed in the upper limb on the paralyzed side after the application of rTMS, while no significant change was observed in the upper limb on the nonparalyzed side (Fig. 2.18) [43].

This suggests that in poststroke upper limb hemiparesis, a pathological increase in the excitability of motor neurons controlling the upper limb on the paralyzed side can be improved. In other words, spasticity can be improved by applying low-frequency rTMS on the nonlesional hemisphere.

Furthermore, there is already a growing body of evidence that the motor function of the upper limb after stroke can be improved by rTMS. Based on our study, we consider that a reduction in spasticity partly contributes to the mechanism of the improvement. We expect that clinically applicable therapeutic intervention for spasticity will be conducted in the future, such as rTMS to enhance the excitability of the affected hemisphere.

6 Neuroimaging Studies of Patients with Upper Limb Hemiparesis

It is believed that rTMS directly influences the cerebral cortex to improve cerebral plasticity. In fact, however, it is still unclear how rTMS and rehabilitation influence plasticity and the functional reorganization of the cerebral cortex. Nonetheless, there are several reports which studied how rTMS and rehabilitation influence on the cerebral blood flow and measured the regional cerebral blood flow (rCBF) using near-infrared spectroscopy (NIRS), single photon emission computed tomography (SPECT), positron emission tomography (PET), and other tools.

In this section, we will introduce some of these reports and describe our own report in which the effects were studied on the basis of a change in rCBF measured by SPECT after performing the 15-day protocol of rTMS and intensive OT during hospitalization (NEURO-15).

A. Report in Which rTMS Was Performed and the Change in rCBF Was Measured by NIRS

Hada et al. [44] measured the blood flow and aerobic metabolism of the cerebral cortex in 12 healthy right-handed subjects using NIRS during and after the performance of rTMS. rTMS was applied on the primary motor area of the left hemisphere controlling the right FDI muscle using a figure-8 coil. Simulation was given 10 times at 0.5 Hz, or 2 Hz and the intensity was 80 % or 120 % of the motor threshold at rest. NIRS probes were placed on the inside edge of the figure-8 coils at 3 cm intervals, and measurement was carried out directly under the stimulation site by the coils. As a result, during and after rTMS stimulation, reduction in the concentration of total hemoglobin (total-Hb) and oxygenated hemoglobin (oxy-Hb) as well as an increase in the concentration of deoxygenated hemoglobin (deoxy-Hb) were observed at stimulation intensities of both 80 % and 120 %. However, Hada et al. said that the mechanism remained unclear.

B. Report in Which rTMS Was Performed and the Change in rCBF Was Measured by SPECT

There are several studies that applied rTMS to healthy subjects and investigated the change in rCBF. One example is a study by Okabe et al. [45], who applied rTMS on the primary motor cortex of the left hemisphere in five healthy subjects and measured rCBF by ^{99m}Tc-ethyl cysteine dimmer (^{99m}Tc-ECD) SPECT. Okabe et al. used figure-8 coils and performed monophasic rTMS (1 Hz, 60 pulses/minute) below the motor threshold. Sham stimulation (fictitious stimulation) was also applied as a control. Radioactive isotopes were injected during stimulation, and the obtained SPECT imaging results were evaluated by using statistic parametric mapping (SPM) 99. As a result, an increase in rCBF was observed in the contralateral (right) cerebellum (Fig. 2.19) [45], while a decrease in rCBF was observed in the primary motor cortex, superior parietal lobule, inferior parietal lobule, dorsal and ventral premotor cortex, and supplementary motor area of the contralateral cerebrum (Fig. 2.20) [45].

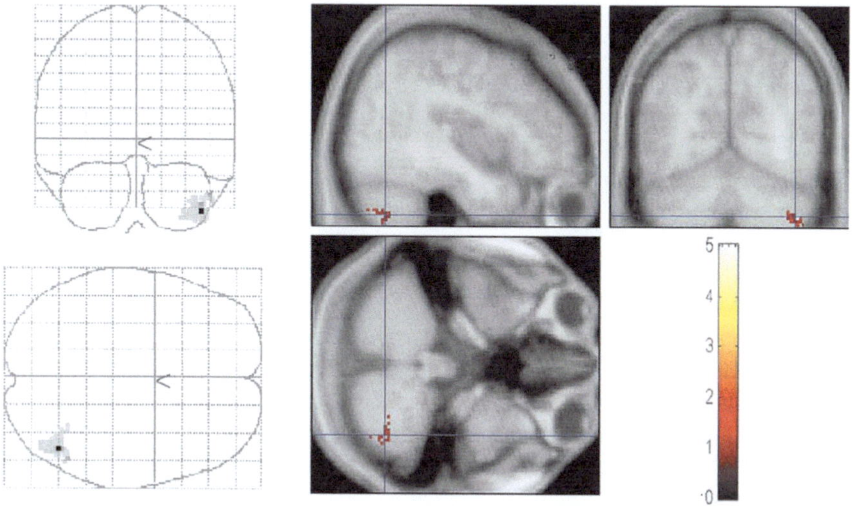

Fig. 2.19 Areas where rCBF increased. The areas where rCBF increased during rTMS on the primary motor cortex of the left hemisphere in comparison with those during the sham stimulation are shown. rCBF increased in the lateral portion of the right posterior cerebellar hemisphere, which is located on the opposite side of the rTMS applied area

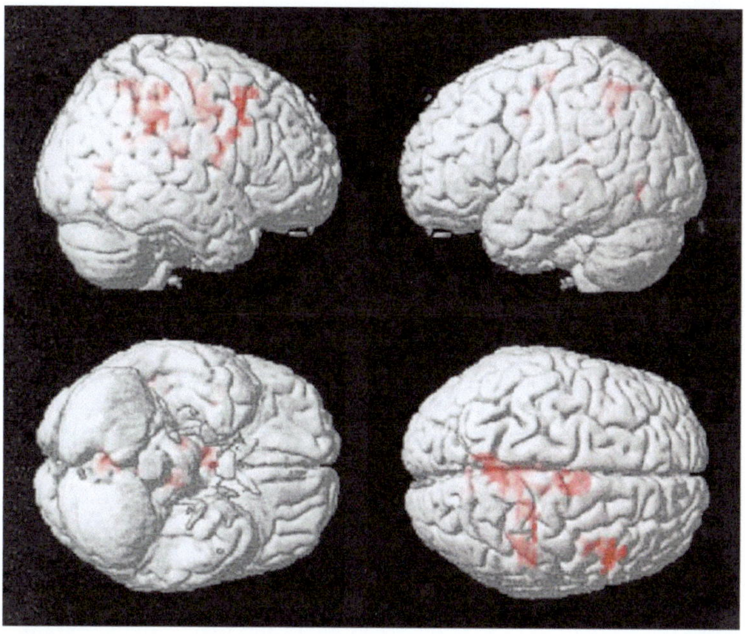

Fig. 2.20 Areas where rCBF reduced. During rTMS on the primary motor cortex of the left hemisphere, a significant decrease in rCBF was observed in the primary motor cortex (M1) including the hand and finger area, the dorsal premotor cortex (dPM), the ventral premotor cortex (vPM), the inferior parietal lobule (IPL) including supramarginal gyrus (Brodmann's area 40), part of the superior parietal lobule (SPL) and the supplementary motor area (SMA) of the right hemisphere. In the left hemispheric imaging, no significant rCBF changes were seen except a few areas over which rCBF decreases in the right hemisphere were projected through the brain

Based on these results, Okabe et al. concluded that low-frequency rTMS at almost same intensity as the motor threshold brings out a change in rCBF. It seems that the cerebellar hemisphere changes its activity in parallel with that of the contralateral primary motor cortex due to strong facilitatory connections between these two areas. Generally, a parallel change in rCBF is commonly known as crossed cerebellar diaschisis.

They consider that the decrease in rCBF in the primary motor cortex of the right hemisphere showed an interhemispheric inhibitory effect via the corpus callosum caused by activation of the primary motor cortex of the left hemisphere and the decrease in rCBF in the right parietal lobe, premotor cortex, and supplementary motor area indicated some secondary effects.

The dynamics of activation of neural activity are usually similar to that of an increase in rCBF and metabolism; however, an increase in rCBF in the motor cortex can be seen when neural activity is suppressed [46]. Therefore, their changes do not necessarily occur in a parallel manner. They mentioned that changes in neural activity may occur even when no change in blood flow was observed. The rCBF reflects the energy consumption, namely, metabolic activity of the vertebral cortex induced by the excitability or inhibitory synaptic activity of the cerebral cortex.

The effects of rTMS on the cortex are a mix of the excitatory and inhibitory neural firings, namely, the synaptic activities [47]. An increase in blood flow means a reduction in physiological activity of the cerebral cortex when it was caused by increased activity of inhibitory synapses.

On the other hand, Hosono et al. [48] made a comparison between monophasic and biphasic rTMS. They performed monophasic rTMS at 0.2 Hz and biphasic rTMS at 1 Hz, with 250 pulses for each, on the left premotor cortex of 7 healthy right-handed subjects (mean age $\pm$ SD: 32.7 $\pm$ 10.7 years old) using a figure-8 coil. Before and after each rTMS, SPECT was carried out and was tested by SPM2. The resultant increase in rCBF was observed at the stimulation site and its adjacent left frontal lobe (Brodmann's area 6) after monophasic stimulation at 0.2 Hz as well as in the left occipital lobe and right parietal lobe after the biphasic stimulation at 1 Hz. No increase was observed in the motor cortex (Fig. 2.21, Table 2.18) [48]. They said that, when applied to the premotor cortex, monophasic rTMS is more useful than biphasic rTMS. The possible reasons for the increase in rCBF in areas distant from the stimulation site are either that when biphasic stimulation at 1 Hz was applied the distant areas were influenced via corticocortical connections [49] or the stimulation is transmitted through the corpus callosum [45].

Relatively few studies have used rTMS for treatment purposes; however, Marcondes et al. [50] performed rTMS in tinnitus patients with normal hearing and performed SPECT examination before and after the stimulation. They randomized 19 patients into either the rTMS at 1 Hz group or the sham stimulation group. As control groups, subjects with normal hearing and patients with tinnitus received rTMS. Stimulation was given on the left temporal-parietal cortex for 5 days. ^{99m}Tc-ECD SPECT imaging was performed before and 14 days after rTMS and a comparison made of the Z score for each voxel before and after the stimulation by the *T*-test. As a result, a decrease in neuronal activity was observed in the left inferior temporal gyrus of the rTMS group.

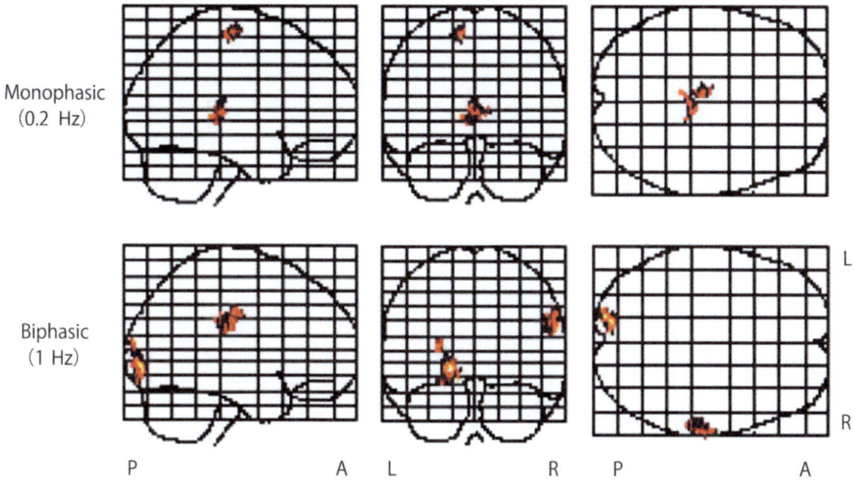

Fig. 2.21 Changes in rCBF by monophasic and biphasic rTMS. Figures shown by maximum intensity projection (MIP). They show the areas where rCBF increased after monophasic and biphasic rTMS on the premotor cortex

Table 2.18 Regional CBF increase after monophasic 0.2 Hz and biphasic 1 Hz rTMS over premotor cortex[a]

Group A	**Condition of rTMS application**	**Brain area**	**Talairach coordinate**			**Z score**
			x	*y*	*z*	
	Monophasic (0.2 Hz)	Left thalamus	0	−23	12	5.03
		Left frontal lobe (Brodmann's area 6)	−8	−11	58	4.27
	Biphasic (1 Hz)	Left occipital lobe (Brodmann's area 17)	−16	−84	−1	4.51
		Left occipital lobe (Brodmann's area 17)	63	−16	−6	3.99

Adapted from Ref. [48]

[a]Talairach coordinates and Z-scores of the sites which showed the maximum value are shown

C. Report in Which Intensive Rehabilitation Was Performed and Changes in rCBF Were Measured by SPECT

There is an interesting report that studied the changes in rCBF by performing SPECT before and after intensive rehabilitation. Könönen et al. [51] studied 12 chronic patients who were recruited after 6 months from the onset of cerebral infarction [mean age: 48 years old, mean time from onset: 36 months (7–132 months)].

Könönen et al. introduced the CIMT defined in the EXCITE study [52], which forces patients to use the paretic upper limb for 2 weeks (Fig. 2.22) [51], and measured rCBF at rest before and 2 weeks after the intervention by using ^{99m}Tc-ECD SPECT.

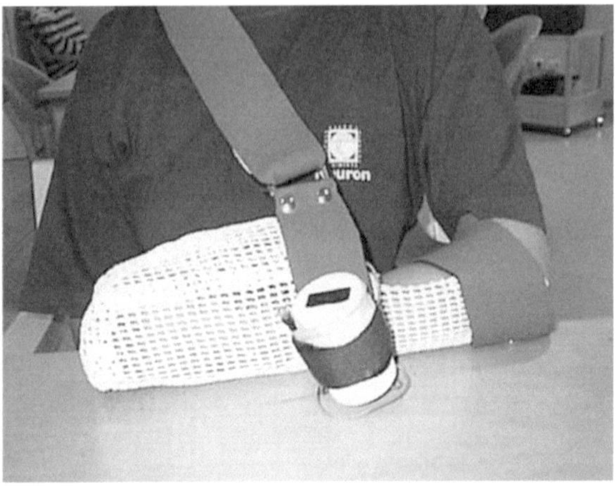

Fig. 2.22 A lightweight sling to constrain the hand-finger and upper limb on the non-paralyzed side. The accompanying watch can detect the patient's body temperature and measure how long he/she has worn the sling [51]

rCBF was tested by using SPM99 and MATLAB®. As a result, increased blood flow was observed in the precentral gyrus of the frontal lobe (Brodmann's area 6) and the superior frontal gyrus of the frontal lobe (Brodmann's area 10) in the affected hemisphere, in the superior frontal gyrus of the frontal lobe (Brodmann's area 6) and the cingulate gyrus (Brodmann's area 31) in the unaffected hemisphere, and on both sides of the cerebellum, while decreased blood flow was observed in the lingual gyrus (Brodmann's area 18) in the affected hemisphere (Fig. 2.23, Table 2.19) [51]. In the unaffected hemisphere, decreased blood flow was observed in the middle frontal gyrus of the frontal lobe (Brodmann's area 8 and 10), the fusiform gyrus of the temporal lobe (Brodmann's area 20), and the inferior temporal gyrus (Brodmann's area 37).

It is known that the superior frontal gyrus integrates information from multiple sensory organs and becomes prepared for movements, while the cingulate gyrus receives signals directly from the primary motor area. The cerebellum has a role in coordinating skilled voluntary movements and is involved in regulating muscle tone and posture. In CIMT, increased blood flow was observed in the area associated with the motion control over the affected side.

D. Report in Which Finger-Tapping Movement Was Performed and Changes in rCBF Were Measured by PET

There is a report that examined changes in rCBF by using PET. Carey et al. [53] investigated the correlation of the evaluation results of upper limb motor function and changes in rCBF measured by PET in nine right-handed stroke patients (seven men, mean age ± SD: 72.0 ± 9.8 years old). Carey et al. assessed the upper limb motor function by ARAT twice: at 2 to 7 weeks after stroke onset (subacute phase) and at 6 months after onset, and they used PET to measure the rCBF when the

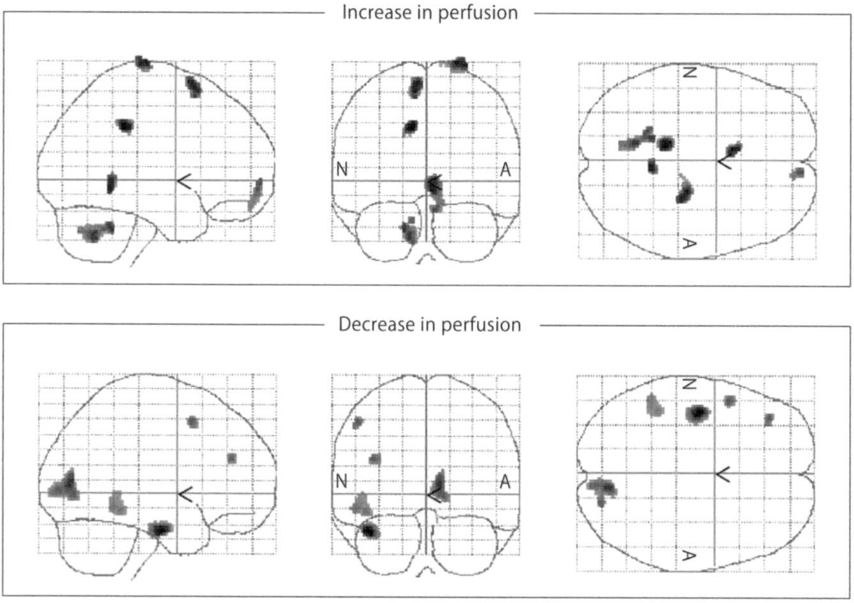

Fig. 2.23 Changes in perfusion by CIMT. The cerebral areas with changed perfusion are shown. The diagrams in the *upper row* show the area where perfusion increased and the diagrams in the *bottom row* show the areas where perfusion decreased. The letter As in the figures show the affected hemisphere and the letter Ns show the non-lesional hemisphere (Adapted from Ref. [51])

Table 2.19 The cerebral areas with changed perfusion in SPECT after two weeks of CIMT

Anatomical area	Perfusion change[a]	Brodmann's area	Size (voxels)	Talairach coordinates[a]			*z*-score[c]
				x	*y*	*z*	
Superior frontal gyrus	+	10	54	8	60	−5	2.97
	+	6	65	−8	18	56	3.24
Precentral gyrus	+	6	67	22	−18	76	3.28
Cingulate gyrus	+	31	65	−10	−35	37	3.57
Cerebellum	+	–	120	−16	−46	−26	3.10
	+	–	54	4	−47	−3	3.26
Medial frontal gyrus	–	10	24	−38	40	20	3.34
	–	8	27	−50	12	46	3.24
	–	20	145	−42	−13	−21	4.61
Inferior temporal gyrus	–	37	111	−50	−45	−7	3.00
Lingual gyrus	–	18	187	10	−75	9	3.77

Adapted from Ref. [51]

[a]+ denotes increased perfusion, – denotes decreased perfusion

[b]A negative value on the x-axis in the Talairach's coordinates denotes the unaffected hemisphere, and a positive value denotes the affected hemisphere

[c]z-score of *t*-test

patient does a simple finger-tapping movement. SPM99 was used for the test. The results showed that in the subacute phase, the linear correlation between changes in the upper limb motor function and movement-related rCBF was observed in the supplementary motor area, the cingulate gyrus of both hemispheres, the insular cortex of the unaffected hemisphere, and the small area of the primary sensory motor area of the affected hemisphere. On the other hand, at 6 months after onset, the corresponding regions were limited mainly to the primary sensory motor area of the affected hemisphere spreading beyond the cingulate gyrus. The authors indicated that the recovery of movement was correlated with the decreased activity of the unaffected hemisphere and the increased activity in the primary sensory motor cortex of the affected hemisphere.

E. Our Study Investigating the Development of Functional Reorganization with rTMS and Rehabilitative Intervention Using Neuroimaging Assessment

The combination therapy of low-frequency repetitive transcranial magnetic stimulation (rTMS) over the nonlesional hemisphere and rehabilitation significantly improves the motor function of patients with upper limb hemiparesis after cerebral infarction. We studied the recovery mechanism using a functional magnetic resonance imaging (fMRI) (1). In this study, we conducted medical interventions in 47 patients with upper limb hemiparesis after cerebral infarction through 15-day hospitalization therapy. Before and after the intervention, fMRI was measured under exercise stress and the laterality index calculated by considering the number of the activated voxels of Brodmann's area 4 and 6 (the laterality index ranged from −1 to 1). Among the subjects who were divided into two groups based on fMRI findings before the intervention, a significant increase in the laterality index was observed after intervention in the patient group which showed an activation in both cerebral hemispheres ($n=27$) ($P<0.05$), and the activation shifted to the lesional hemisphere [63]. On the other hand, a significant increase in the activity of the lesional hemisphere was observed in the patient group which showed an activation in only one of the cerebral hemispheres ($n=20$) ($P<0.05$) [63]. It was suggested that the intervention induced the functional cerebral cortex to be restructured, which may have led to the upper limb motor function recovery on the paralyzed side (1).

We also conducted another study with 33 patients with upper limb hemiparesis after stroke. In this study, the relevant cerebrocortical areas were examined before and after the intervention with rTMS and the intensive occupational therapy by considering the correlation of the change in the upper limb motor function and the change in the regional cerebral blood flow (2). We used FineSRT to perform SPECT to measure the regional cerebral blood flow with 99mTc-ECD and measured the blood flow levels in 46 regions corresponding to the individual gyrus which subdivided the region of interest (ROI). In addition, the ROI analysis was conducted over six major Brodmann's areas. The asymmetry indices (AIs) were calculated in 52 regions [64] using the average of the right and left ROI and the correlation examined between the change in the AIs and the differences in the Fugl-Meyer Assessment (FMA) before and after the intervention. As a result, out of the 52 regions, a significant correlation was observed in the superior frontal gyrus and the middle frontal gyrus [64]. It was suggested that the improvement of the upper limb motor function by FMA was associated with the improvement of the regional cerebral blood flow of the superior frontal gyrus and the middle frontal gyrus (2).

F. Our Report in Which rTMS Was Performed and Changes in rCBF Were Measured by SPECT

There have been no studies reporting the effects of rTMS on poststroke patients based on changes in rCBF measured by SPECT. Thus, we examined how our ongoing NEURO-15 influences a patient's brain and has an effect on the plasticity and the functional reconstruction of the cerebral cortex [54].

1) Study Patients

Of the poststroke patients with upper limb hemiparesis who met all the eligibility criteria of NEURO-15, we studied 17 inpatients in our department (Jikei University Hospital) in whom SPECT could be retrospectively performed at the time of admission and at 4 weeks after discharge. The clinical background of the study patients is shown in Table 2.20; the mean age at the time of intervention was 56.0 ± 10.2 years old (23–67 years old) and the mean time from onset to intervention 56.9 ± 39.4 months

Table 2.20 Clinical background of the study patients

Age at the time of intervention (years old)		56.0 ± 10.2
Male/female		12/5
Subtype of stroke	Cerebral infarction	4
	Subcortical hemorrhage	10
	Putaminal hemorrhage	1
	Thalamic hemorrhage	2
Dominant hand/paralyzed hand	Right/right	13
	Right/left	3
	Left/left	1
BRS (median)	Hand-finger	Stage IV
	Upper limb	Stage IV
Time from onset to intervention (months)		56.9 ± 39.4

(17.5–134.3 months). The subtypes of stroke of the study patients included four cerebral infarctions, ten subcortical hemorrhages, one putamen hemorrhage, and two thalamic hemorrhages. The affected area varied from patient to patient; however, none of them brought about obstacles when making an analysis by SPM5. The affected areas included 13 left hemispheres and 4 right hemispheres, or 14 upper limbs on the dominant hand side and 3 upper limbs on the nondominant hand side.

The median BRS at the time of intervention was Stage IV for both the upper limb and hand-finger. This study was conducted with the approval of the ethics committee of our university. We obtained informed consent from all patients.

2) Treatment Protocol

The treatment protocol consisted of the low-frequency rTMS and intensive OT based on the NEURO-15. One session of low-frequency rTMS at 1 Hz lasted for 20 minutes (1200 pulses). The intensive OT as a combination therapy lasted for 120 minutes, which was conducted daily (two sessions daily) except on the morning of the admission day and Sunday. A total of 23 sessions were conducted over 15 days. Similar to NEURO-15, the stimulation site was the primary motor area of the unaffected hemisphere and the intensity set at 90 % of the motor threshold. Upper limb-related items in FMA and the performance time of 15 tasks in WMFT were used to evaluate the upper limb motor function. SPECT and the upper limb motor function test were performed before intervention (immediately after admission and 4 weeks after discharge).

3) Examination and Analysis by SPECT

SPECT examination was performed in patients at rest and with their eyes closed, by using ^{99m}Tc-ethyl cysteine dimmer (^{99m}Tc-ECD) as a tracer. Intravenous 600 MBq of ^{99m}Tc-ECD was administered to patients at rest and with their eyes closed and the images taken 20 minutes later. SPECT was analyzed using SPM5 [55, 56]. After the images of patients whose right hemisphere was affected were inverted, the analysis was performed and all of them considered as left hemisphere lesions. A paired *t*-test was used for an image analysis at the time of admission and 4 weeks after discharge.

4) Results

All 17 study patients completed the 15-day treatment protocol, and no adverse events and adverse reactions were observed during hospitalization. No patient experienced any adverse events or adverse reactions during 4 weeks from discharge. With regard to the changes in the evaluation of upper limb motor function before and after intervention, upper limb-related items in FMA showed a significant increase from 42.76 ± 11.97 points (mean ± SD) to 45.52 ± 11.38 points ($P < 0.001$) and the performance time of 15 tasks in WMFT a significant decrease from 3.18 ± 1.18 to 2.64 ± 1.38 ($P < 0.001$). A significant increase in rCBF was observed in the insular cortex (Brodmann's area 13), the precentral gyrus (Brodmann's area 44), the cerebellum in the affected hemisphere, and the tongue gyrus (Brodmann's area 18) and the cerebellum in the unaffected hemisphere. A decrease in rCBF was observed in the middle frontal gyrus (Brodmann's area 6), the precentral gyrus (Brodmann's area 4), and the posterior central gyrus (Brodmann's area 3) in the unaffected hemisphere (Fig. 2.24). The Talairach coordinates and Z-score of each area are as shown in Table 2.21.

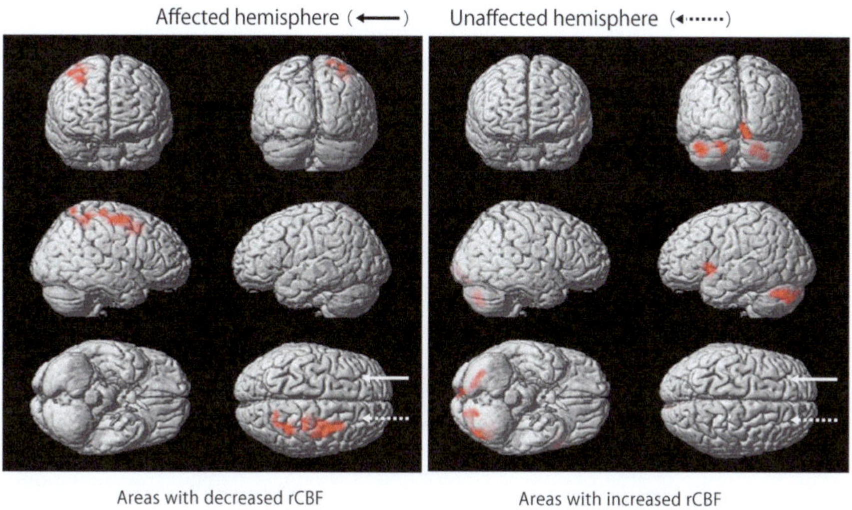

Fig. 2.24 Areas with relative increases and decreases in local cerebral blood flow

Table 2.21 Areas where perfusion changes were observed before and after rTMS intervention

Area of brain	Area of brain	Perfusion change			Brodmann's area	Z score
		x	y	z		
Left insular cortex	+	−40	10	−4	13	5.90
	+	−45	8	1	13	5.41
Left precentral gyrus	+	−54	13	8	44	5.33
	+	−45	−66	−33	–	6.43
Left cerebellum	+	−18	−81	−31	–	6.16
	+	−16	−72	−35	–	5.99
Right lingual gyrus	+	3	−92	−12	18	6.64
	+	4	−85	−13	18	5.97
Right cerebellum	+	6	−80	−19	–	5.75
	+	25	−72	−33	–	6.31
	+	29	−65	−41	–	6.15
Right middle frontal gyrus	–	28	2	45	6	7.62
Right postcentral gyrus	–	20	−32	59	3	7.28
Right precentral gyrus	–	33	−20	52	4	6.73

5) Discussion

Imaging comparison studies before and after CIMT by SPECT, such as the report by Könönen et al. [51] described above, which were conducted to expect changes in the plasticity of the cerebrum, showed an increase in rCBF mainly in the precentral gyrus and the frontal gyrus in the affected hemisphere, while a decrease in rCBF was observed in the medial part, fusiform gyrus, and inferior temporal gyrus of the frontal lobe in the nonlesional hemisphere. This is similar to our research results. Swayne et al. [57] suggested that in chronic stroke the established imbalance of interhemispheric inhibition and additional inhibitory stimulus from the unaffected hemisphere might inhibit the establishment of the plasticity of the affected hemisphere. This study suggested that the increase in rCBF in the precentral gyrus (Brodmann's area 44) and its adjacent insular cortex (Brodmann's area 13) in the affected hemisphere might have meant that low-frequency rTMS and intensive OT relieved the imbalance of interhemispheric inhibition and improved the activity of the affected area and its surrounding area.

Furthermore, in this study, a significant increase in rCBF was observed in the lingual gyrus of the unaffected hemisphere. It delivers visual information from the V1 region of the visual association area to its subregion. In particular, the V2 region is an area where visual information is delivered separately into the dorsal stream and the ventral stream [58] and is a major transit point for visual information.

In particular, the dorsal stream delivers information to the middle temporal gyrus, the premotor area, and the premotor cortex and plays a major role in planning and conducting movements. In other words, the study results suggest that there is a possibility that low-frequency rTMS and the intensive OT brought about a change in rCBF in the cerebrum and the areas that are responsible for planning and conducting movements were activated, which resulted in an increase in rCBF in the lingual gyrus.

One of the limitations of this study was that self-exercise in the intensive OT varied from patient to patient. For this reason, each patient did not necessarily have an improvement in the plasticity of the cerebral cortex in the identical area through exercise. Secondly, this study was not an RCT that included a control group but included the intervention group only. We consider that it is necessary to verify the effects of low-frequency rTMS on rCBF and the effects of the intensive OT on rCBF independently. However, they have yet to be verified because there are problems with patient consent and the number of cases to obtain. In addition, this study had an issue in that the increase in rCBF in the affected hemisphere was observed only in the precentral gyrus and the insular cortex. A previous report indicated that the premotor area and the supplementary motor area may also play an important role in improving plasticity after stroke and in reorganizing the network [59]; however, the same results were not obtained in our study. For this reason as well, we believe that there is a need to examine a larger sample size.

7 Future Challenges

To date, we have worked with more than 1800 patients in our institution and our 9 associated institutions. The effectiveness was demonstrated in the multicenter study including 204 patients described above (p. 35) as well as in the multicenter study including as many as 1008 cases that is currently being submitted. In addition, international research papers are increasingly being published as a result of the sufficient recognition of rTMS as an effective treatment for neurological sequelae of stroke. The future challenges based on the results obtained from NEURO will be described below.

A. Timing to Perform rTMS

Our department started a combination therapy of low-frequency rTMS on the unaffected hemisphere and the unique intensive OT in poststroke patients with upper limb hemiparesis in April 2008, which was called the "six-day protocol." After confirming its safety, we started performing an extended "15-day protocol" named NEURO-15 in April 2009. This is a treatment in which low-frequency rTMS, which has an inhibitory effect of neural activity in local brain areas, is applied on the unaffected hemisphere, which reduces interhemispheric inhibition between the unaffected and the affected hemisphere, makes the affected hemisphere free from inhibition, and leads to a recovery in upper limb motor function. The eligibility criteria of NEURO-15 stipulate that a patient should be enrolled after 1 year from onset. In NEURO, the magnetic stimulation device that is originally not a therapeutic instrument but testing equipment is used as a therapeutic instrument after obtaining a patient's consent as well as the approval of the ethical committee of each institution. We therefore believe that NEURO-15 should be applied only in patients who are in a safer or more stable condition. Consequently, to date, NEURO has been conducted safely as we expected.

However, a report using a functional MRI (fMRI) in the subacute or acute stroke showed that activation of the unaffected hemisphere occurs at 3 months after onset or later [60]. Based on this fact, if rTMS treatment is performed in acute stroke, high-frequency rTMS on the affected hemisphere might be more effective. In fact, Sasaki et al. [61] conducted RCT that included 29 patients who were enrolled within 29 days after onset and divided them into the following 3 groups: high-frequency rTMS of 10 Hz group (1000 pulses in 10 minutes), low-frequency rTMS of 1 Hz group (1800 pulses in 30 minutes), and sham stimulation group. Comparing the results before and after the intervention, both the high-frequency and the low-frequency rTMS groups showed a significant increase in grip strength and tapping number. However, a statistically significant increase compared to the sham stimulation group was observed only in the high-frequency rTMS group (Fig. 2.25) [61].

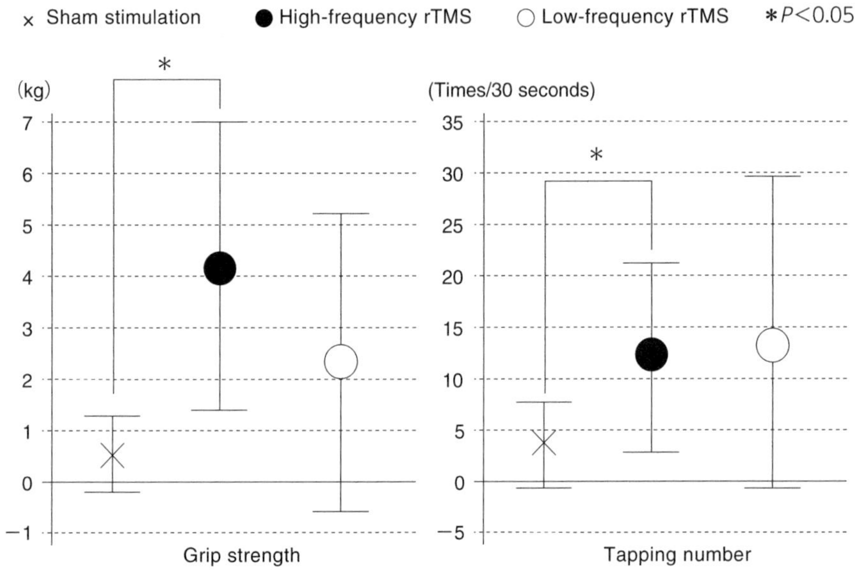

Fig. 2.25 Changes in grip strength and tapping number in three groups before and after intervention. The values are expressed as mean ± SD. Statistical analysis was performed by the unpaired *t*-test [61]

On the other hand, a report showed that stronger interhemispheric inhibition was observed in patients with poorer recovery of motor function after stroke [62]. Therefore, it is speculated that low-frequency TMS on the unaffected hemisphere is optimal for patients beyond 3 months from onset and whose motor function has been poorly recovered. We believe that the optimal timing of rTMS intervention and eligible patients for rTMS treatment should be determined based on its therapeutic properties after further consideration of rTMS.

B. Parameters of rTMS

For the challenges, see Chap. 7, section "Clinical Introduction of Other Stimulation Modalities" (p. 164).

C. Challenges with Rehabilitation Programs

Symptoms of patients with stroke range widely, therefore it is important to offer an approach appropriate for the symptoms as well as rehabilitation appropriate for changes in neural function brought about by rTMS. For this purpose, we must accurately assess the patient's physical function and higher brain function and further understand the effects of rTMS. Based on these factors, we should understand the patient's needs and demands and set up a strategy to achieve them.

What is important here is which should be emphasized, namely, "the upper limb function exercise" including gross motor and dexterity movements or "the combined movements exercise" including bimanual operations such as ADL and object manipulation training. Even if the upper limb motor function is sufficient, an ideal pattern of target movement cannot be immediately achieved if the exercise program has not been adequately established. In addition, if a patient with insufficient upper limb function works on a target movement exercise, he/she may not be able to achieve an ideal pattern of target movement since an exercise program with compensatory patterns is followed. Therefore, as shown in Fig. 2.26, it is necessary to adjust the balance between "the upper limb function exercise" and "the combined movements exercise" along with the motor function improvement due to rehabilitation.

However, if a patient continues to avoid use of the upper limb on the paralyzed side in ADL because of its immobility, the activation of the affected hemisphere can be inhibited due to learned nonuse. Therefore, such a patient should use the upper limb on the paralyzed side in ADL as much as possible from an earlier stage, such as putting the upper limb on the paralyzed side on the table during a meal and cleaning the floor with a rag using both hands, as well as rolling over and getting up without using the handrail if the trunk is unstable (including movements starting from the paralyzed side).

It has already been reported that NEURO-15 enables a patient to reacquire not only the upper limb motor function on the paralyzed side but also movements in ADL. There are no reports to date that showed movements in ADL can be reacquired by conducting rTMS alone; however, there is a possibility that rTMS can enhance motion learning. Thus, further studies should be conducted in the future.

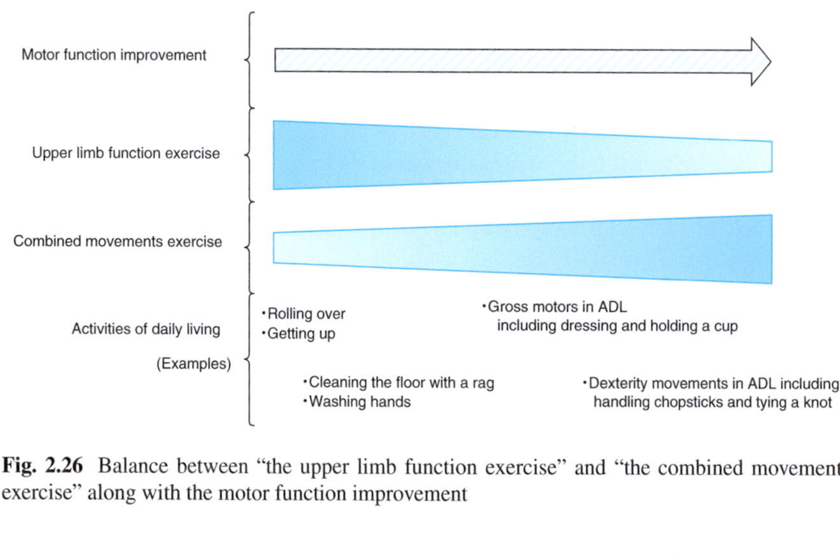

Fig. 2.26 Balance between "the upper limb function exercise" and "the combined movements exercise" along with the motor function improvement

D. Disparity of the Technical Level among Therapists and Differences of Rehabilitation Approach

Rehabilitation techniques greatly vary depending on the individual patient as well as the institution. The directions of rehabilitation also differ from each other: some focus on the functional improvement of the upper limb on the paralyzed side, while others focus on the acquisition of ADL movements by the nonparalyzed side. However, NEURO is a new treatment that can improve the upper limb function on the paralyzed side in a short period of time, which to date has been considered unable to be improved. Therefore, in NEURO, it is necessary to accurately evaluate a patient's function, which continually changes from day to day, and to adjust the rehabilitation approach depending on the situation. Therapists and physicians must fully understand the mechanism of NEURO and maintain advanced skills and high aspirations.

All institutions currently conducting NEURO are our associated institutions that had received and passed through the training at Jikei University School of Medicine. Medical staff at our department continue to provide them with direct instruction. Thus, these nine institutions can provide almost the same effect to patients receiving NEURO. Moreover, we have a system for exchanging information as needed online, and to share data. We also hold an annual workshop, which enables us to continue to develop through friendly competition among institutions.

In recent years, facilities other than our associated institutions have started applying a rehabilitation approach by reference to NEURO, although a lack of understanding about NEURO, ambiguous inclusion criteria, an obvious skill shortage of therapists, and other issues remain. We therefore decided to introduce a training system in consultation with our associated institutions for the purpose of obtaining the same effect in any facility.

This training is intended for institutions that will be introducing NEURO-15 in the future and consists of the direction of rehabilitation, basic learning about the disease, rehabilitation knowledge and skills, and the study of rTMS. After an institution completes the training, we take into account the reported results for a certain number of patients and determine if we can approve them as a NEURO providing institution. We believe that this process enables all NEURO providing institutions to improve their technical level and enables patients to receive treatment at the same level at any institution. Currently, the training session for NEURO-15 introduction is being held at Jikei University Hospital (Tokyo, Japan).

E. Application to Sensory Disturbance

Quite a few patients who wish to receive NEURO-15 have sensory disturbance. Sensory information is transmitted to the brain through the spinal cord and other nerves after sensory receptors receive not only visual and auditory information but also information input from a certain part of the body. Information transmitted to the brain is integrated with a variety of information such as the current physical and mental condition, memory information, and the property of an object and leads to cognition and action. This process enables a person to keep the body in balance consciously or unconsciously, to understand the name of an object, and to move an object to where it should be.

Patients with stroke are often directed to work on upper limb motor function training with an awareness of the joint movement, muscle tone, and others. This training helps to increase the various kinds of selected information about the site and the movement, to activate the brain, and to facilitate the activity of the neural sprouting and unmasking, which results in improvement of upper limb motor function. With a sensory disturbance, however, information cannot be properly input, or if it has been input, it cannot be perceived, and the patient cannot be aware of the movement, which brings about sensory ataxia or motor learning impairment. With regard to the therapeutic effect of NEURO-15, it has been reported that patients with sensory disturbance show poorer improvement in the upper limb motor function on the paralyzed side compared to patients without sensory disturbance. In addition, patients cannot be aware of the therapeutic effects even after they have been obtained and cannot easily feel a sense of satisfaction. We think there is a need to review the stimulation site, intensity, and methods when performing rTMS in patients with sensory disturbance or to consider an entirely different approach in the future.

F. Application to Higher Cerebral Dysfunction

In recent years, researchers have started studying a new treatment using rTMS for higher brain dysfunction. Our department has been working on aphasia in particular and has performed inpatient treatment that is a combination treatment of low-frequency rTMS and speech training. However, research into attention disorders, memory impairment, apraxia, and agnosia remains insufficient.

Higher brain dysfunction varies depending on the part of the brain that has been injured. For example, when the parietal lobe is damaged, ideational apraxia, constructional apraxia, and hemispatial neglect (hemispatial agnosia) may occur. Aphasia, memory impairment, and auditory agnosia may occur when the temporal lobe is injured; visual agnosia, prosopagnosia, and Balint's syndrome may occur when the occipital lobe is injured; and executive dysfunction, attention disorders, and affective disorders may occur when the frontal lobe is injured. That is, since the symptoms vary depending on the injured area, it is necessary to determine which area is injured and to understand which pathway is inhibited by the injury, such as in commissural, association, or projection fibers, and which area is being used to compensate it.

Based on the understanding of the process described above, rTMS can finally be performed. Ultimately, however, it is extremely hard to determine which area is being used for a compensatory function. While it is possible to examine it using fMRI or other methods, a patient must exactly understand the examiner's instructions and perform the procedure. Quite a few patients with higher brain dysfunction have difficulty in maintaining attention or cannot exactly perform a movement as directed because of impaired comprehension. Therefore, we consider that it is necessary to investigate techniques that enable us to grasp the compensatory area and the stimulating methods of rTMS even in these patients. Higher brain dysfunction is not yet properly understood outside the healthcare sector, and patients may be forced to leave their employment and suffer from a mental illness such as depression because of troubles in social relationships or at work. In addition, most insurance policies do not cover higher brain dysfunction as a special case of premium payment exemption. This creates difficulties for countless patients with higher brain dysfunction. Future research is imperative so that rTMS can be a ray of hope for patients with higher brain dysfunction.

References

1. Shinohara Y, Ogawa S, et al. Japanese guidelines for the management of stroke. Tokyo: Kyowa Kikaku; 2009. p. 308–12. Japanese.
2. Langhorne P, Coupar F, Pollock A. Motor recovery after stroke; a systematic review. Lancet Neurol. 2009;8:741–54.
3. Duncan PW, Goldstein LB, Matchar D, et al. Measurement of motor recovery after stroke. Outcome assessment and sample size requirements. Stroke. 1992;23:1084–9.
4. Jørgensen HS, Nakayama H, Raaschou HO, et al. Stroke. Neurologic and functional recovery the Copenhagen Stroke Study. Phys Med Rehabil Clin N Am. 1999;10:887–906.
5. Liepert J, Bauder H, Wolfgang HR, et al. Treatment-induced cortical reorganization after stroke in humans. Stroke. 2000;31:1210–6.
6. Dong Y, Dobkin BH, Cen SY, et al. Motor cortex activation during treatment may predict therapeutic gains in paretic hand function after stroke. Stroke. 2006;37:1552–5.
7. Hsu WY, Cheng CH, Liao KK, et al. Effects of repetitive transcranial magnetic stimulation on motor functions in patients with stroke; a meta-analysis. Stroke. 2012;43:1849–57.
8. Wassermann EM. Risk and safety of repetitive transcranial magnetic stimulation; report and suggested guidelines from the international workshop on the safety of repetitive transcranial magnetic stimulation, June 5–7, 1996. Electroencephalogr Clin Neurophysiol. 1998;108:1–16.
9. Wolf SL, Winstein CJ, Miller JP, et al. Effect of constraint-induced movement therapy on upper extremity function 3 to 9 months after stroke; the EXCITE randomized clinical trial. JAMA. 2006;296:2095–104.
10. Brunnstrom S. Movement therapy in hemiplegia. New York: Harper and Row; 1970.
11. Fugl-Meyer AR, Jääskö L, Leyman I, et al. The post-stroke hemiplegic patient. 1. A method for evaluation of physical performance. Scand J Rehabil Med. 1975;7:13–31.
12. Van der Lee JH, Beckerman H, Lankhorst GJ, et al. The responsiveness of the Action Research Arm test and the Fugl-Meyer Assessment scale in chronic stroke patients. J Rehabil Med. 2001;33:110–3.
13. Hsieh CL, Hsueh IP, Chiang FM, et al. Inter-rater reliability and validity of the action research arm test in stroke patients. Age Ageing. 1998;27:107–13.
14. Carroll D. A quantitative test of upper extremity function. J Chronic Dis. 1965;18:479–91.
15. Lyle RC. A performance test for assessment of upper limb function in physical rehabilitation treatment and research. Int J Rehabil Res. 1981;4:483–92.

16. Takahashi K, Domen K, Sano K, et al. Reliability and validity of the Motor Activity Log in Japan. J Jpn Occup Ther Assoc. 2009;28:628–36. Japanese.
17. Ishikawa A, Kakuda W, Taguchi K, et al. The reliability and validity of a new subjective assessment scale for poststroke upper limb hemiparesis, the Jikei Assessment Scale for Motor Impairment in Daily Living. Tokyo Jikei Med J. 2010;125:159–67. Japanese.
18. Hara Y. Therapy for hemiplegic upper extremity in stroke patients. Gen Rehabil. 2009;37:711–7. Japanese.
19. Miyaguchi H. "Current" neurorehabilitation in occupational therapy: from the standpoint of cognitive exercise therapy. Jpn J Occup Ther. 2009;43:333–42. Japanese.
20. Kakuda W, Abo M, Shimizu M, et al. Combination treatment of low-frequency repetitive transcranial magnetic stimulation and intensive occupational therapy for upper limb hemiparesis after stroke: clinical results in more than a thousand patients. Jpn J Stroke. 2013;35:274–80.
21. Fuzaro AC, Guerreiro CT, Galetti FC, et al. Modified constraint-induced movement therapy and modified forced-use therapy for stroke patients are both effective to promote balance and gait improvements. Rev Bras Fisioter. 2012;16:157–65.
22. Mancebo A, Molier T, González B, et al. Acute oral, pulmonary and intravenous toxicity/pathogenicity testing of a new formulation of Bacillus thuringiensis var israelensis SH-14 in rats. Regul Toxicol Pharmacol. 2011;59:184–90.
23. Van Vliet PM, Wulf G. Extrinsic feedback for motor learning after stroke; what is the evidence? Disabil Rehab. 2006;28:831–40.
24. Nakama S. Self-exercise for stroke patients at home. J Phys Ther. 2008;25:390–6. Japanese.
25. Taub E, Uswatte G, Mark VW, et al. The learned nonuse phenomenon: implications for rehabilitation. Eura Medicophys. 2006;42:241–56.
26. Morris DM, Taub E, Mark VW. Constraint-induced movement therapy: characterizing the intervention protocol. Eura Medicophys. 2006;42:257–68.
27. Law M, Baptiste S, McColl M, et al. The Canadian occupational performance measure; an outcome measure for occupational therapy. Can J Occup Ther. 1990;57:82–7.
28. Welmer AK, von Arbin M, Widén Holmqvist L, et al. Spasticity and its association with functioning and health-related quality of life 18 months after stroke. Cerebrovasc Dis. 2006;21:247–53.
29. Kakuda W, Abo M, Kobayashi K, et al. Anti-spastic effect of low-frequency rTMS applied with occupational therapy in post-stroke patients with upper limb hemiparesis. Brain Inj. 2011;25:496–502.
30. Sommerfeld DK, Eek EU, Svensson AK, et al. Spasticity after stroke: its occurrence and association with motor impairments and activity limitations. Stroke. 2004;35:134–9.
31. Watkins CL, Leathley MJ, Gregson JM, et al. Prevalence of spasticity post stroke. Clin Rehabil. 2002;16:515–22.
32. Lance JW. Symposium synopsis. Spasticity; disordered motor control. Chicago: Year Book Medical; 1980. p. 485–94.
33. Brown P. Pathophysiology of spasticity. J Neurol Neurosurg Psychiatry. 1994;57:773–7.
34. Sehgal N, McGuire JR. Beyond Ashworth. Electrophysiologic quantification of spasticity. Phys Med Rehabil Clin N Am. 1998;9:949–79.
35. Tanaka R. The neural mechanisms of spasticity: revisited. Jpn J Rehabil Med. 1995;32:97–105. Japanese.
36. Bohannon RW, Smith MB. Interrater reliability of a modified Ashworth scale of muscle spasticity. Phys Ther. 1985;67:206–7.
37. Kimura J, Kohara N. A study guide of nerve conduction study and electromyogram. 2nd ed. Tokyo: Igaku-Shoin; 2010. Japanese.
38. Tsai KH, Yeh CY, Chang HY, et al. Effects of a single session of prolonged muscle stretch on spastic muscle of stroke patients. Proc Natl Sci Counc Repub China B. 2001;25:76–81.
39. Burke D, Gandevia SC, McKeon B. The afferent volleys responsible for spinal proprioceptive reflexes in man. J Physiol. 1983;339:535–52.
40. Centonze D, Koch G, Versace V, et al. Repetitive transcranial magnetic stimulation of the motor cortex ameliorates spasticity in multiple sclerosis. Neurology. 2007;68:1045–50.

41. Wupuer S, Yamamoto T, Katayama Y, et al. F-wave suppression induced by suprathreshold high-frequency repetitive transcranial magnetic stimulation in poststroke patients with increased spasticity. Neuromodulation 24 Oct 2012.
42. Málly J, Dinya E. Recovery of motor disability and spasticity in post-stroke after repetitive transcranial magnetic stimulation (rTMS). Brain Res Bull. 2008;76:388–95.
43. Kondo T, Kakuda W, Yamada N, et al. Effect of low-frequency rTMS on motor neuron excitability after stroke. Acta Neurol Scand. 2013;127:26–30.
44. Hada Y, Abo M, Kaminaga T, et al. Detection of cerebral blood flow changes during repetitive transcranial magnetic stimulation by recording hemoglobin in the brain cortex, just beneath the stimulation coil, with near-infrared spectroscopy. Neuroimage. 2006;32:1226–30.
45. Okabe S, Hanajima R, Ohnishi T, et al. Functional connectivity revealed by single-photon emission computed tomography (SPECT) during repetitive transcranial magnetic stimulation (rTMS) of the motor cortex. Clin Neurophysiol. 2003;114:450–7.
46. Strafella AP, Paus T. Cerebral blood-flow changes induced by paired-pulse transcranial magnetic stimulation of the primary motor cortex. J Neurophysiol. 2001;85:2624–9.
47. Loo CK, Sachdev PS, Haindl W, et al. High (15Hz) and low (1Hz) frequency transcranial magnetic stimulation have different acute effects on regional cerebral blood flow in depressed patients. Psychol Med. 2003;33:997–1006.
48. Hosono Y, Urushihara R, Harada M, et al. Comparison of monophasic versus biphasic stimulation in rTMS over premotor cortex: SEP and SPECT studies. Clin Neurophysiol. 2008;119:2538–45.
49. Siebner HR, Filipovic SR, Rowe JB, et al. Patients with focal arm dystonia have increased sensitivity to slow-frequency repetitive TMS of the dorsal premotor cortex. Brain. 2003;126(Pt 12):2710–25.
50. Marcondes RA, Sanchez TG, Kii MA, et al. Repetitive transcranial magnetic stimulation improve tinnitus in normal hearing patients: a double-blind controlled, clinical and neuroimaging outcome study. Eur J Neurol. 2010;17:38–44.
51. Könönen M, Kuikka JT, Husso-Saastamoinen M, et al. Increased perfusion in motor areas after constraint-induced movement therapy in chronic stroke; a single-photon emission computerized tomography study. J Cereb Blood Flow Metab. 2005;25:1668–74.
52. Winstein CJ, Miller JP, Blanton S, et al. Methods for a multisite randomized trial to investigate the effect of constraint-induced movement therapy in improving upper extremity function among adults recovering from a cerebrovascular stroke. Neurorehabil Neural Repair. 2003;17:137–52.
53. Carey LM, Abbott DF, Egan GF, et al. Motor impairment and recovery in the upper limb after stroke; behavioral and neuroanatomical correlates. Stroke. 2005;36:625–9.
54. Hara T, Kakuda W, Kobayashi K, et al. Regional Cerebral Blood Flow (rCBF) after low-frequency Repetitive Transcranial Magnetic Stimulation (rTMS) combined with intensive occupational therapy for upper limb hemiplegia after stroke: a study using single photon emission computed tomography. Jpn J Rehab Med. 2013;1:36–42. Japanese.
55. Frinston KJ, Holmes A, Worsley KJ, et al. Statistical parametric maps in functional imaging; a general linear approach. Hum Brain Mapp. 1995;2:189–210.
56. Ashburner J, Friston KJ. Nonlinear spatial normalization using basis functions. Hum Brain Mapp. 1999;7:254–66.
57. Swayne OB, Rothwell JC, Ward NS, et al. Stages of motor output reorganization after hemispheric stroke suggested by longitudinal studies of cortical physiology. Cereb Cortex. 2008;18:1909–22.
58. Kravitz DJ, Saleem KS, Baker CI, et al. A new neural framework for visuospatial processing. Nat Rev Neurosci. 2011;12:217–30.
59. Ward NS, Brown MM, Thompson AJ, et al. Neural correlates of motor recovery after stroke; a longitudinal fMRI study. Brain. 2003;126:2476–96.
60. Marshall RS, Perera GM, Lazar RM, et al. Evolution of cortical activation during recovery from corticospinal tract infarction. Stroke. 2000;31:656–61.

61. Sasaki N, Mizutani S, Kakuda W, et al. Comparison of the effects of high- and low-frequency repetitive transcranial magnetic stimulation on upper limb hemiparesis in the early phase of stroke. J Stroke Cerebrovasc Dis. 2013;22:413–8.
62. Reis J, Swayne OB, Vandermeeren Y, et al. Contribution of transcranial magnetic stimulation to the understanding of cortical mechanisms involved in motor control. J Physiol. 2008;586:325–51.

Additional References

63. Yamada N, Kakuda W, Senoo A, Kondo T, Mitani S, Shimizu M, et al. Functional cortical reorganization after low-frequency repetitive transcranial magnetic stimulation plus intensive occupational therapy for upper limb hemiparesis: evaluation by functional magnetic resonance imaging in poststroke patients. Int J Stroke. 2013;8(6):422–9.
64. Takekawa T, Kakuda W, Uchiyama M, Ikegaya M, Abo M. Brain perfusion and upper limb motor function: a pilot study on the correlation between evolution of asymmetry in cerebral blood flow and improvement in Fugl-Meyer assessment score after rTMS in chronic post-stroke patients. J Neuroradiol. 2014;41(3):177–83.

Chapter 3
rTMS for Poststroke Aphasia

1 Pathology and Current Status of the Treatment

A. Classification of Aphasia

Aphasia is defined as "condition characterized by impaired expression and comprehension of language representation resulted from post-lingual damage to the language center of the cerebrum due to some causes." While articulation disorders are caused by impaired exophasia (motor speech disorder), aphasia is considered to correspond to impaired endophasia (impairment of the language center of the cerebrum). The most frequent cause of aphasia is stroke, which accounts for approximately 90 % of all cases of aphasia, and followed by head injury. The major subtypes of stroke are a middle cerebral artery stroke and putaminal hemorrhage.

In more than 90 % of right-handed individuals and 60–70 % of left-handed individuals the language center is located in the left hemisphere, and the inferior frontal gyrus of the frontal lobe (Brodmann's areas 44 and 45), which is called Broca's area, and the superior temporal gyrus of the temporal lobe (Brodmann's areas 41 and 42), which is called Wernicke's area, are considered to correspond to the language center (Fig. 3.1).

Aphasia is classified into some types depending on the language function that is impaired. In case of damage to the Broca's area, typically patients present with "motor aphasia (Broca's aphasia)," namely, their auditory comprehension is maintained but spontaneous speech and handwriting are impaired, whereas in case of damage to the Wernicke's area, spontaneous speech is fluent but auditory comprehension is impaired, and patients present with "sensory aphasia (Wernicke's aphasia)," which is associated with paraphasia.

Other relatively common types of aphasia include global aphasia following extensive damage to the frontal lobe (both auditory comprehension and spontaneous

M. Abo, W. Kakuda, *Rehabilitation with rTMS*,
DOI 10.1007/978-3-319-20982-1_3

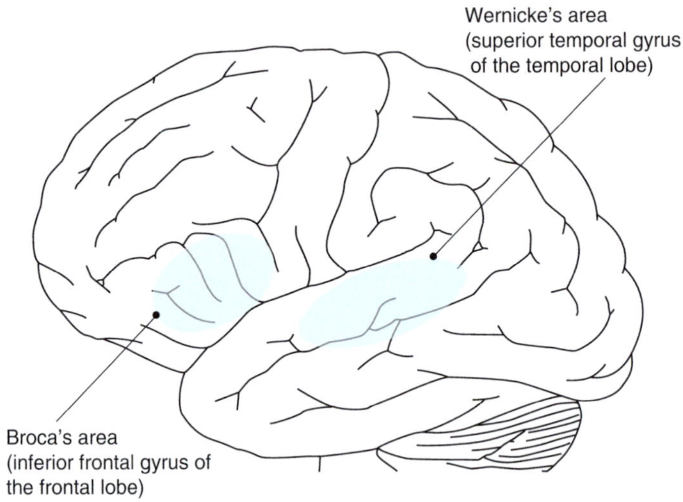

Fig. 3.1 Location of the language center. The language center is located in the frontal and temporal lobe of the human brain

speech are severely impaired), amnesic aphasia (the ability to name objects is severely impaired), and conduction aphasia (speech repetition is severely impaired).

B. Aphasia and Rehabilitation

The history of rehabilitation for the treatment of poststroke aphasia is by no means short, and training methods such as Schuell's systematic stimulation and facilitation method, the deblocking method proposed by Weigl, and functional reorganization method proposed by Luria are widely known [1]. In the "Japanese Guidelines for the Management of Stroke 2009," [2] "intensive and professional speech and language therapy (ST) for the treatment of aphasia from an early time point after stroke onset" is recommended with Grade B evidence. However, at present no firm evidence on the beneficial effects of these training methods has been accumulated yet.

On the other hand, based on our vast experience with the treatment of patients with aphasia, we have the impression that "compared to motor paralysis, in case of post-stroke patients with aphasia, the potential for recovery is sustained over a long period of time." More specifically, in the case of poststroke aphasia, the therapeutic window for rehabilitation intervention is wide, and we think that even in patients of chronic aphasia for several years after stroke, there is a possibility that language function will recover by conducting appropriate rehabilitation. This opinion has become the basis of our attempts to treat chronic poststroke aphasia through active therapeutic intervention.

2 Low-Frequency rTMS of the Right Frontal Lobe

In fact, the first time that rTMS was reported to have been used as therapeutic intervention of poststroke patients with aphasia was by the group around Naeser et al. [3] from Boston University. However, prior to this attempt by Naeser et al., Belin et al. [4] and Rosen et al. [5] had reported overactivity in the right frontal lobe of patients with aphasia resulting from impairment of the left frontal lobe and had interpreted this overactivity in the right frontal lobe as a maladaptive response that causes an extensive interhemispheric inhibition of the left hemisphere, thus preventing the compensation of language function through the left hemisphere.

Based on these reports, Naeser et al. [3] thought that it might be possible to reduce the extensive interhemispheric inhibition of the left hemisphere by means of low-frequency rTMS stimulation, which has an inhibitory effect on the unusually high activation levels in the right frontal lobe, and that this eventually might lead to the release of the left frontal lobe from interhemispheric inhibition, thus activating its compensatory role in language function (Fig. 3.2). In 2005 Naeser et al. [6] reported about a pilot study that involved four poststroke patients with motor aphasia resulting from lesions in the left frontal lobe, due to a stroke 5–11 years ago.

Naeser et al. treated these patients by applying 1-Hz low-frequency rTMS every day for 20 minutes (a total of 1200 pulses) over a period of 10 days to the inferior frontal gyrus of the right frontal lobe, which is located just contralateral to the Broca's area. As a result, it was found that directly after 10 days of rTMS the patients were able to recall the name of more objects than before treatment, and also

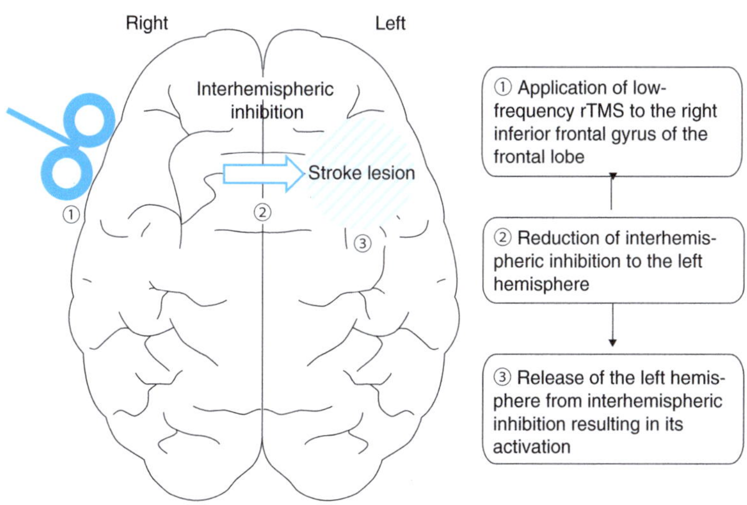

Fig. 3.2 Treatment concept of Naeser et al. The reduction of the interhemispheric inhibition to the left hemisphere by suppressing overactivity in the right hemisphere leads to the release of the left hemisphere that takes in a compensatory role in language function from inhibition, which in turn results in its activation

other improvements were observed, such as that the time required to recall the name of these objects had shortened. Moreover, these improvements were confirmed to have maintained also 8 months after conducting rTMS.

This study suggested that the application of low-frequency rTMS to the right frontal lobe for the treatment of aphasia resulting from lesions in the left frontal lobe might become a therapeutic intervention, and also hereafter there were continuous reports that confirmed the usefulness thereof.

Barwood et al. [7] divided 12 patients with aphasia resulting from lesions in the left frontal lobe into 2 groups. One group was treated with low-frequency rTMS to the right frontal lobe, and the other group was treated with sham stimulation to the same site for 10 days. As a result, it was found that in the low-frequency rTMS group language functions such as the ability to name objects had significantly improved compared to the sham stimulation group. Moreover, Weiduschat et al. [8] compared in a similar fashion the degree of improvement of language functions between a group treated with low-frequency rTMS to the right frontal lobe and a sham stimulation group. As a result, after 2 weeks of stimulation the improvement of language functions was significantly better in the low-frequency rTMS group. In addition, in the report by Weiduschat et al. positron emission tomography (PET) scans taken over time confirmed that neural activity in the left hemisphere had increased as a result of low-frequency rTMS to the right frontal lobe.

3 Importance of the Right Hemisphere for Compensating Language Function

Low-frequency rTMS to the right frontal lobe for the treatment of aphasia resulting from impairment of the left frontal lobe as proposed by Naeser et al. [3, 6] is based on the assumption that primarily the left hemisphere plays an important role in the compensation of language function. However, in fact, there are also several reports that demonstrate that the right hemisphere is involved in the compensation of language function.

Ohyama et al. [9] demonstrated by use of PET that in patients with motor aphasia resulting from impairment of the left frontal lobe the degree of language function recovery was correlated with the degree of right frontal lobe activation. Moreover, Abo et al. [10] showed by use of functional MRI (fMRI) that in patients in whom a favorable recovery of language functions was observed also an activation of the right hemisphere was seen. Moreover, Richter et al. [11] announced similar findings in a study that used fMRI.

In view of these clinical reports, we think that there is a possibility that in case of aphasia resulting from impairment of the left frontal lobe the site that can compensate language function is not necessarily limited to the left hemisphere but that depending on the patient rather the right hemisphere plays a central role in the compensation of language functions. Therefore, high activation levels in the right hemisphere, which are seen when the left hemisphere was damaged, are not necessarily a maladaptive response but depending on the patient can be interpreted to indicate "new activity that can be used for the compensation of language functions."

4 Application of Functional MRI in Therapeutic Approach to Aphasia

Not only when applying rTMS for the treatment of aphasia but also when applying rTMS for the treatment of other neurological sequelae of stroke, it is important that the neural activity of the site that compensates impaired functions is activated. Considering the diversity of sites that can compensate language function in patients with aphasia resulting from impairment of the left frontal lobe, it is desirable to sort out which site can compensate language function before applying rTMS treatment in patients with aphasia.

For instance, it is believed that the possibility cannot be ruled out that the compensation of language functions might become inhibited, if low-frequency rTMS is applied to a brain area that compensates language function, and that as a result language functions aggravate. At present, however, there are no special clinical findings that suggest sites that compensate language function in patients with aphasia, and it is also not possible to evaluate such sites by common head CT or MRI. Therefore, we considered that it might be possible to evaluate sites that compensate language function in patients with aphasia by use of fMRI images that were obtained while the patient performed verbal tasks and devised a therapeutic approach of rTMS, which is conducted based on such images.

It is a treatment concept in which sites that showed activity on fMRI images that were obtained while the patient performed verbal tasks are considered compensatory sites of language function and in which the compensation of language function is promoted by reducing the interhemispheric inhibition of the activated site by applying low-frequency rTMS to the contralateral hemisphere [12]. In short, for motor aphasia resulting from impairment of the left frontal lobe, in patients with activity in the left hemisphere on fMRI images that were obtained while the patient performed verbal tasks, low-frequency rTMS is applied to the inferior frontal gyrus of the right frontal lobe, and in contrast, in patients with activity in the right hemisphere on fMRI images that were obtained while the patient performed verbal tasks, low-frequency rTMS is applied to the inferior frontal gyrus of the left frontal lobe (Fig. 3.3).

There is a notable report on this method that was also published by Naeser et al. [13] According to Naeser et al., in patients in whom fMRI imaging of verbal tasks prior to the application of rTMS confirmed activity not only in the right but also in left hemisphere, not only language functions such as naming recovered after application of low-frequency rTMS to the right frontal lobe, but also increased activation of the left hemisphere was confirmed on fMRI images. On the other hand, in patients in whom fMRI images prior to the application of rTMS only confirmed activity in the right hemisphere, through the application of low-frequency rTMS to the right

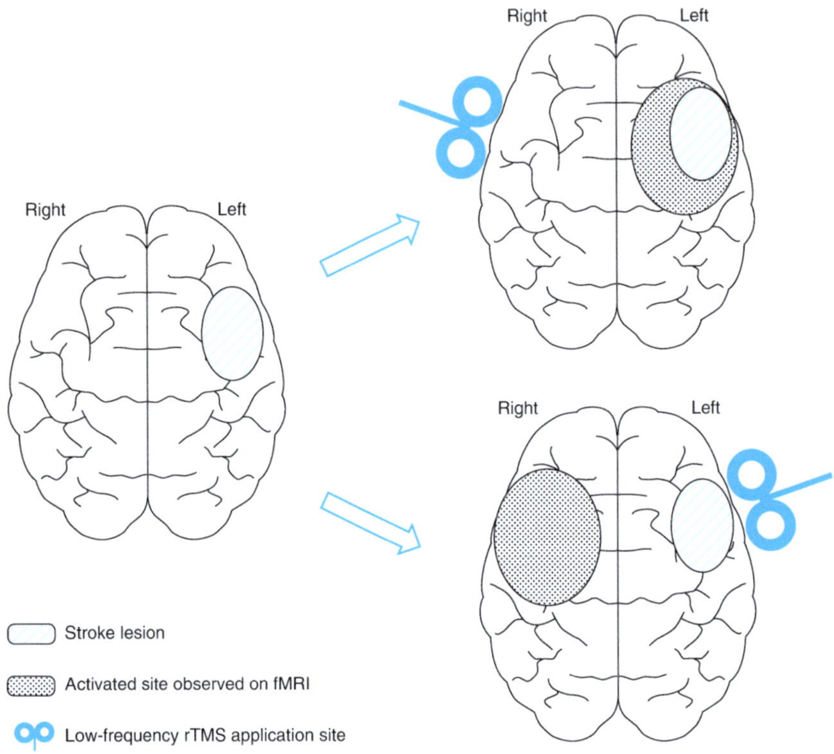

Fig. 3.3 Application site for low-frequency rTMS determined based on fMRI findings. Low-frequency rTMS is applied over the hemisphere contralateral to the activated site on fMRI images

frontal lobe neither a recovery of language functions nor increased activity was observed at any site. Therefore Naeser et al. concluded that "it is unlikely to achieve positive effects through the application of low-frequency rTMS to the right hemisphere in patients in whom no activity was observed in the left hemisphere on fMRI images taken prior to the application of rTMS," and we think that this supports our concept."

5 Protocol of Low-Frequency rTMS in Combination with Intensive Speech and Language Therapy

In a cooperative study with the Division of Radiological Science, Faculty of Health Science, Tokyo Metropolitan University, which has excellent expertise in fMRI imaging, we conduct rTMS for the treatment of poststroke aphasia resulting from lesions in the left frontal lobe since 2007. This therapy is only conducted in those patients who visited our outpatient department (Department of Rehabilitation, Jikei

University Hospital) because they wish to undergo this treatment and who fulfill the eligibility criteria. Our treatment policy is to determine the site that is suitable for treatment, based on the results of fMRI images that were obtained while the patient performed verbal tasks, and then to perform low-frequency rTMS in combination with intensive ST on consecutive days after the patient was hospitalized at our department (Fig. 3.4). The actual protocol is described below.

A. Eligibility Criteria

The current eligibility criteria are the same as those listed in Table 3.1, such as the contraindications for rTMS in the guidelines suggested by Wassermann [14]. However, these criteria are considered to be only provisional, and it should be noted that these criteria might be revised in the future.

B. fMRI Images of Verbal Tasks

For the evaluation of compensatory sites of language function, fMRI images that are obtained while the patient is performing verbal tasks are taken at least 4 weeks prior to hospitalization for undergoing rTMS treatment.

All MRI images are obtained by use of 3.0-Tesla equipment, which enables echo-planar imaging. fMRI is performed using gradient-echo echo-planar imaging, and imaging parameters are set as follows: slice thickness 5 mm, field of view (FOV) 230 mm, time of repetition (TR) 5000 ms, time to echo (TE) 35 ms, flip angle 90°, and matrix size 128×128.

One fMRI examination session is performed under two conditions, namely, in performing speech repetition tasks and in a resting state. Speech repetition task is to repeat aloud the short words that can be heard every 5 minutes via earphone. However, before performing speech repetition tasks, we confirmed whether the

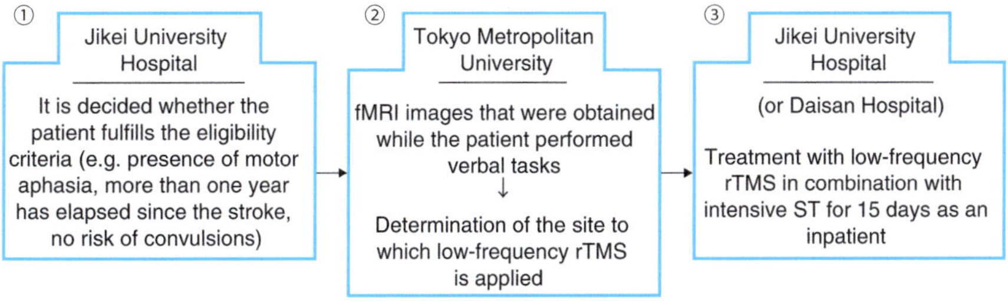

Fig. 3.4 Procedure of the application of rTMS for the treatment of aphasia at our department. In patients who fulfill the eligibility criteria, fMRI is conducted while the patient performs verbal tasks, and the site to which low-frequency rTMS is applied is determined

Table 3.1 Eligibility criteria for the applications of rTMS for the treatment of aphasia

1.	Presenting mild-to-moderate motor aphasia due to stroke (e.g., ability, at least, to speak short sentences comprising two to four Japanese words, to repeat aloud nouns frequently used in daily living settings, to understand and follow simple verbal commands, to communicate with others in daily living settings)
2.	Age at application of treatment between 18 and 80 years
3.	The latency between the onset of stroke and application of treatment is more than 12 months
4.	History of a single stroke only (no bilateral cerebrovascular lesion)
5.	No apparent cognitive impairment (other than aphasia)
6.	No apparent changes in language function at least three months prior to the application of treatment (despite of speech rehabilitation)
7.	No active systemic physical or mental illness requiring medical management
8.	No pathological conditions known to be contraindications for rTMS in the guide-lines suggested by Wassermann (e.g., intracranial metals, cardiac pacemaker, pregnancy)
9.	No recent history of seizure (documented epileptic discharge on recent electroencephalography or current use of antiepileptic medications for the prevention of seizure)

As of December, 2012

patient who was examined was able to repeat correctly most of the words that he or she heard.

Moreover, simultaneously, for the accurate positioning of the activated site that was superimposed on fMRI images, also horizontal and coronal T1-weighted images were taken. The imaging parameters for T1-weighted images were set as follows: slice thickness 2 mm, FOV 240 mm, TR 26 ms, TE 2.4 ms, flip angle 80°, and matrix size 256×256. fMRI images were analyzed by use of statistical parametric mapping 2 (SPM2) software implemented in MATLAB® for the analysis of brain imaging data. Analyzed images were displayed in such a way that they were superimposed on horizontal and coronal T1-weighted images. Sites with an increase in local blood flow (*P* values of 0.01 or less) were shown as significant activated site, and the *T* value (indicates the degree of increase in blood flow) of each activated site was automatically calculated. Furthermore, the hemisphere that contained the activated site with the highest *T* value was considered to be the "compensatory language function hemisphere."

Figure 3.5 represents typical examples of fMRIs in which activation is seen in the left and right hemisphere, respectively.

C. Application of Low-Frequency rTMS

Low-frequency rTMS stimulation of 1 Hz is performed by use of MagPro R30 and a figure-8 coil (both manufactured by MagVenture). One session lasts 20 minutes, and thus during one session 1, 200 pulses of 1 Hz are applied. At first we decided to

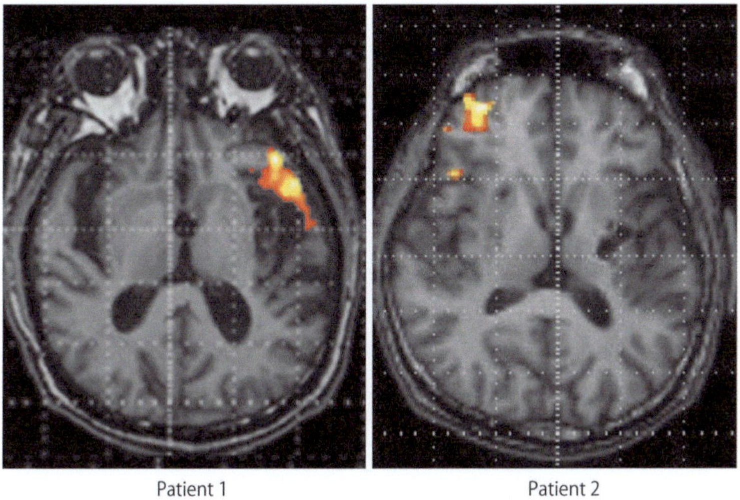

Fig. 3.5 fMRI images that were obtained while the patient performed verbal tasks. Activation can be seen in the left frontal lobe for patient 1 and in the right frontal lobe for patient 2

set the site contralateral to "the site that showed the strongest activation on fMRI" as stimulation site; however, it was extremely complicated to work out a method pursuant to this idea (MRI images were taken after marking the site, e.g., with a coin, and the stimulation site was determined by correcting deviations between the target site and the position of the coin). Moreover, some voiced the opinion that "if it were possible to accurately determine to which hemisphere rTMS should be applied, then it would not be necessary to stimulate the site exactly contralateral to the maximum activated site."

Therefore, at present the inferior frontal gyrus of the frontal lobe in the hemisphere contralateral to "the hemisphere that contains the most activated site on fMRIs" is set as the stimulation site (in the left hemisphere this corresponds to the Broca's area, and in the right hemisphere this corresponds to the region contralateral to the Broca's area). Furthermore, for determining the position of the inferior frontal gyrus of the frontal lobe we apply the International 10–20 system.

Previously, Homan et al. [15] and Okamoto et al. [16] examined in detail the correlation between International 10–20 system electrode placement sites and cerebral localization. As a result, both research groups concluded that the F7 region (left hemisphere) and F8 region (right hemisphere) correspond to the inferior frontal gyrus of the frontal lobe. Therefore, in patients in whom activation was observed in the left hemisphere on fMRI we use the F8 region as stimulation site, and in patients in whom activation was observed in the right hemisphere on fMRI we use the F7 region as stimulation site (Fig. 3.6).

MagPro R30 is equipped with an arm with which the stimulation coil is fixated, and because this arm is very strong, as long as the patient does not move markedly,

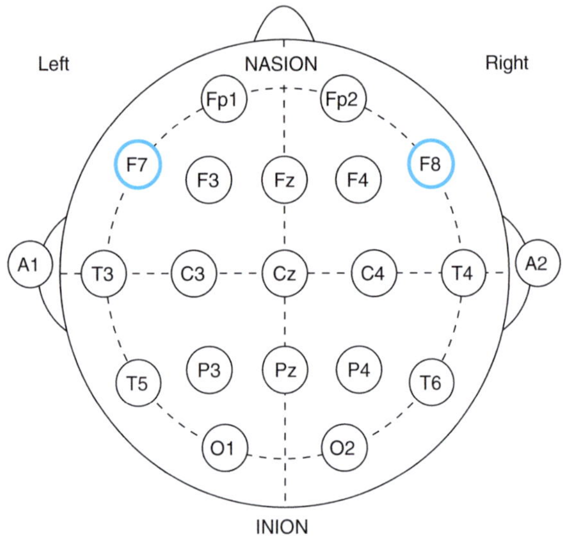

Fig. 3.6 F7 and F8 regions of the International 10–20 system. The F7 and F8 regions correspond to the inferior frontal gyrus of the frontal lobe

it will rarely happen that the stimulation site will be misaligned. However, during rTMS the physician should always stay by the patient, and frequently check whether the stimulation site has become misaligned, and also watch out for adverse events or adverse reactions. We thought to put a small circular sticker on the stimulation site once it was determined, or to mark the stimulation site on the skin by use of a marker pen (p. 124), so that at the next treatment session rTMS could be applied to the same site. Regardless to which hemisphere rTMS is applied, intensity was set at 90 % of the minimum intensity (motor threshold) measured with which MEP can be induced in the left (nonparalyzed side) thenar muscles of upper limb (Table 3.2).

D. Treatment Protocol During Hospitalization

rTMS treatment for the treatment of aphasia is performed in combination with intensive ST and requires hospitalization for a period of 15 days (Table 3.3). In principle, except for the day of hospitalization/discharge and Sundays, every day twice low-frequency rTMS is performed for 20 minutes, and twice intensive ST is performed for 60 minutes. Intensive ST is a one-on-one training with a speech therapist that is individually designed according to the severity and impaired functions of the patient, but essentially this program focuses on the strengthening of speech modalities.

This program mainly comprises, for instance, "training by use of sentences to describe the contents" about presented pictures or cartoons, "training to repeat aloud" the words or sentences the therapist said, and "training to dictate" as listening to short words or sentences. Language functions were assessed at least twice, namely, prior to hospitalization and at time of discharge, by use of the standard

Table 3.2 An example of rTMS treatment for the treatment of aphasia[a]

Coil used	Figure-8 coil
Site	Non-lesional hemisphere (frontal lobe inferior frontal gyrus)
Intensity	90 % of motor threshold
Frequency	Low-frequency rTMS (1 Hz)
Duration	1 session lasting 20 minutes (1200 pulses), once or twice daily
No. of days of hospitalization	15 days

[a]The actual therapeutic regimen is adjusted by each institution
As of December, 2012

language test of aphasia (SLTA) and the Japanese version of western aphasia battery (WAB). In the "Japanese Guidelines for the Management of Stroke 2009" [2] the use of SLTA as well as the Japanese version of WAB is recommended with Grade B evidence.

E. Results

Here, we introduce the results from the pilot study of this combination treatment in 12 patients with motor aphasia resulting from left frontal lobe stroke conducted between 2009 and 2011 [17].

This study included six patients each with intracerebral hemorrhage of the left putamen and with left middle cerebral artery infarction. Mean age at the time of treatment was approximately 55 years old, and approximately 38 months had passed between stroke onset and intervention. fMRI images that were obtained while the patient performed verbal tasks revealed the left hemisphere was activated in nine patients and the right hemisphere in three patients. Therefore, in nine patients low-frequency rTMS was applied to the F8 region, and in three patients low-frequency rTMS was applied to the F7 region (Table 3.4) [17]. As described above, each patient was hospitalized for 15 days and during this period underwent the treatment with 20 minutes of low-frequency rTMS in combination with 60 minutes of ST twice daily.

As a result, we found that the rate of correct answers obtained when testing naming in the SLTA test or repetition in the WAB test had significantly improved. Moreover, also a tendency of improved correct answer rates for other items (speech repetition and handwriting in the SLTA test) was observed (Table 3.5) [17]. Based on these results, we speculated that the application of low-frequency rTMS had increased the plasticity of compensatory sites of language function shown on fMRI and that in combination with intensive ST the functional reconstruction of language functions had been promoted, and we considered that it would be useful to check this over time (before and after treatment) by functional brain imaging such as fMRI or PET. In addition, we think that the results of this study confirmed the safety of this combination treatment; however, there is a possibility that the duration

Table 3.3 Example of the hospitalization of rTMS treatment for the treatment of aphasia[a]

	Thur	Fri	Sat	Sun	Mon to Sat	Sun	Mon and Tues	Wed	Thur
Morning	Admission	Evaluation at admission	Low-frequency rTMS (20 minutes)	No treatment	Low-frequency rTMS (20 minutes)	No treatment	Low-frequency rTMS (20 minutes)		Discharge
			One-to-one training (60 minutes)		One-to-one training (60 minutes)		One-to-one training (60 minutes)		
Afternoon	Pre-treatment evaluation	Low-frequency rTMS (20 minutes)			Low-frequency rTMS (20 minutes)		Low-frequency rTMS (20 minutes)	Post-treatment evaluation	
		One-to-one training (60 minutes)			One-to-one training (60 minutes)		One-to-one training (60 minutes)		

[a]An example of being hospitalized on Thursday
The actual hospitalization schedule is adjusted by each institution
As of December, 2012

Table 3.4 Clinical characteristics of studied patients

No	Gender	Age at intervention (years)	Time between stroke onset and intervention (m)	Type of stroke	Site of lesion	Hemisphere including the most activated area	rTMS application site
1	M	49	31	Intracerebral hemorrhage	Left putamen	Left	F8
2	M	58	27	Intracerebral hemorrhage	Left putamen	Left	F8
3	M	57	51	Cerebral infarction	Left middle cerebral artery territory	Left	F8
4	M	61	15	Cerebral infarction	Left middle cerebral artery territory	Left	F8
5	F	56	30	Cerebral infarction	Left middle cerebral artery territory	Left	F8
6	M	49	41	Cerebral infarction	Left middle cerebral artery territory	Left	F8
7	M	59	33	Intracerebral hemorrhage	Left putamen	Left	F8
8	M	46	19	Cerebral infarction	Left middle cerebral artery territory	Left	F8
9	F	44	28	Intracerebral hemorrhage	Left putamen	Left	F8
10	M	58	15	Intracerebral hemorrhage	Left putamen	Right	F7
11	M	66	115	Intracerebral hemorrhage	Left putamen	Right	F7
12	M	62	48	Cerebral infarction	Left middle cerebral artery territory	Right	F7

Reference [17]

Table 3.5 Changes in outcome measures by intervention

Outcome measures		Correct answer rate (%)		P value
		Pre-intervention	Post-intervention	
SLTA	Naming	77.5 ± 18.3	84.6 ± 15.3	<0.05
	Repetition	75.1 ± 17.9	78.4 ± 15.0	0.082
	Writing	70.4 ± 34.6	73.3 ± 30.1	0.22
Japanese version of WAB	Repetition	68.7 ± 27.0	75.7 ± 25.9	<0.05

Reference [17]

of intervention (duration of hospitalization) or the duration of rTMS were not optimal, and therefore these points require further examination.

6 Future Challenges

To this point, we have described the therapeutic application of rTMS for the treatment of poststroke motor aphasia; however, until now there are almost no reports on the therapeutic application of rTMS for the treatment of sensory aphasia.

As described above, motor aphasia typically results from impairment of the frontal lobe, and sensory aphasia results from impairment of the temporal lobe. There are attempts also to treat patients with sensory aphasia who have lesions in the temporal lobe by applying rTMS to the frontal lobe, similar to the treatment of motor aphasia; however, we remain dubious as to whether this is appropriate. In fact, the neural connections between both hemispheres do not only correspond one to one, and therefore it is expected that there is also a possibility that the application of rTMS to the frontal lobe may affect the contralateral temporal lobe; however, the impact thereof might not be sufficient.

Therefore, we thought that for the treatment of sensory aphasia resulting from temporal lobe lesions, rTMS should also be applied to the temporal lobe (although there is not much evidence for this concept). We also thought that, particularly when the left hemisphere is affected, the superior temporal gyrus of the temporal lobe that corresponds to the Wernicke's area should be used as the stimulation site and actually selected CP5 (left hemisphere) and CP6 (right hemisphere), which according to the International 10–20 system correspond to the superior temporal gyrus as stimulation sites. Recently, the application of rTMS treatment is not ruled out even for the treatment of sensory aphasia, and a "therapeutic rTMS concept that does not only take into consideration of findings prior to the application of rTMS, but also of the type of aphasia" has been started. More specifically, based on fMRI findings and the type of aphasia (clinical findings) patients are divided into four groups, as shown in Fig. 3.7, and for each type rTMS application site is selected. In summary patients are divided into the following groups:

(i) For motor aphasia with activation in the left hemisphere on fMRI, low-frequency rTMS is applied to the F8 region (right hemisphere).

(ii) For motor aphasia with activation in the right hemisphere on fMRI, low-frequency rTMS is applied to the F7 region (left hemisphere).
(iii) For sensory aphasia with activation in the left hemisphere on fMRI, low-frequency rTMS is applied to the CP6 region (right hemisphere).
(iv) For sensory aphasia with activation in the right hemisphere on fMRI, low-frequency rTMS is applied to the CP5 region (left hemisphere).

The outcome of this new treatment concept so far is generally favorable [18]. Moreover, we have consistently used low-frequency rTMS for the treatment of patients with aphasia, but we believe that also approaches should be tested that use high-frequency rTMS instead. More specifically, this is a treatment concept that tries to facilitate the neural activity of compensatory sites of language function directly by applying high-frequency rTMS to compensatory sites of language function that were determined by fMRI. Eventually it will become necessary to compare the effects of approaches that use this kind of high-frequency rTMS and approaches that use low-frequency rTMS as we do on the improvement of language functions.

From the results of our initiatives we expect that similar to other neurological sequelae of stroke, the recovery of poststroke aphasia can be facilitated by performing intensive ST after the brain's plasticity was increased by use of rTMS. However,

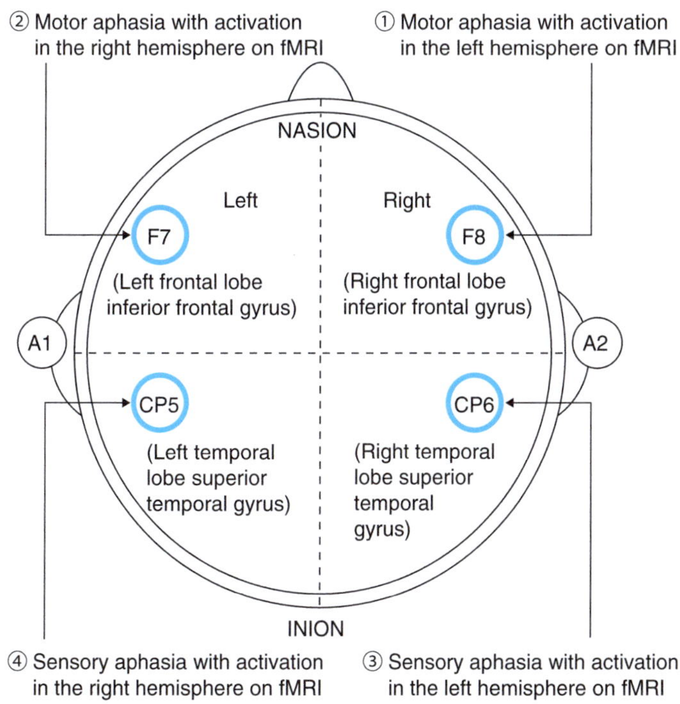

Fig. 3.7 Application site of rTMS based on fMRI findings and the type of motor aphasia, low-frequency-rTMS is applied to the frontal lobe. On the other hand, in case of sensory aphasia, low-frequency rTMS is applied to the temporal lobe

an important point with regard to the treatment of aphasia by use of rTMS is the determination of the site that can compensate language function before applying rTMS. We sincerely hope that in the future the usefulness of conservative language rehabilitation will increase through the appropriate application of rTMS treatment.

References

1. Kakuda W, Abo M. Speech therapy (aphasia): cutting-edge treatment of neurological disorders 2012–2014. Nankodo; 2011. pp. 388–91. Japanese.
2. Shinohara Y, Ogawa S, et al. Japanese guidelines for the management of stroke. Tokyo: Kyowa Kikaku; 2009. p. 308–12. Japanese.
3. Naeser MA, Martin PI, Nicholas M, et al. Improved naming after TMS treatments in a chronic, global aphasia patient-care report. Neurocase. 2005;11:182–93.
4. Belin P, Van Eeckhout P, Zilbovicius M, et al. Recovery from nonfluent aphasia after melodic intonation therapy; a PET study. Neurology. 1996;47:1504–11.
5. Rosen HJ, Ojemann JG, Ollinger JM, et al. Comparison of brain activation during word retrieval done silently and aloud using fMRI. Brain Cogn. 2000;42:201–17.
6. Naeser MA, Martin PI, Nicholas M, et al. Improved picture naming in chronic aphasia after TMS to part of Broca's area; an open-protocol study. Brain Lang. 2005;93:95–105.
7. Barwood CH, Murdoch BE, Whelan BM, et al. Improved language performance subsequent to low-frequency rTMS in patients with chronic non-fluent aphasia post-stroke. Eur J Neurol. 2011;18:935–43.
8. Weiduschat N, Thiel A, Rubi-Fessen I, et al. Effects of repetitive transcranial magnetic stimulation in aphasic stroke; a randomized controlled pilot study. Stroke. 2011;42:409–15.
9. Ohyama M, Senda M, Kitamura S, et al. Role of the nondominant hemisphere and un-damaged area during word repetition in poststroke aphasics: a PET activation study. Stroke. 1996;27:897–903.
10. Abo M, Senoo A, Watanabe S, et al. Language-related brain function during word repetition in post-stroke aphasics. Neuroreport. 2004;15:1891–4.
11. Richter M, Miltner WH, Straube T. Association between therapy outcome and right hemisphere activation in chronic aphasia. Brain. 2008;131:1391–401.
12. Kakuda W, Abo M, Kaito N, et al. Functional MRI-based therapeutic rTMS strategy for aphasic stroke patients; a case series pilot study. Int J Neurosci. 2010;120:60–6.
13. Naeser MA, Martin PI, Treglia E, et al. Research with rTMS in the treatment of aphasia. Restor Neurol Neurosci. 2010;28:511–29.
14. Wassermann EM. Risk and safety of repetitive transcranial magnetic stimulation; report and suggested guidelines from the international workshop on the safety of repetitive transcranial magnetic stimulation, June 5–7, 1996. Electroencephalogr Clin Neurophysiol. 1998;108:1–16.
15. Homan RW, Herman J, Purdy P. Cerebral location of international 10–20 system electrode placement. Electroencephalogr Clin Neurophysiol. 1987;66:376–82.
16. Okamoto M, Dan H, Sakamoto K, et al. Three-dimensional probabilistic anatomical cranio-cerebral correlation via the international 10–20 system oriented for transcranial functional brain mapping. Neuroimage. 2004;21:99–111.
17. Kakuda W, Abo M. Functional MRI-based strategy of therapeutic rTMS application; a novel approach for post-stroke aphasic patients. Intellectual and developmental disabilities. Rijeka: In Tech; 2012.
18. Abo M, Kakuda W, Watanabe M, et al. Effectiveness of low-frequency rTMS and intensive speech therapy in poststroke patients with aphasia: a pilot study based on evaluation by fMRI in relation to type of aphasia. Eur Neurol. 2012;68:199–208.

Chapter 4
rTMS for Poststroke Dysphagia

1 Pathology and Current Status of the Treatment

A. Etiology and Pathology of Dysphagia

Besides organic disorders of the oral cavity and pharynx, dysphagia is caused by neuromuscular dysfunction, which can also be associated with aging. Furthermore, stroke-related dysphagia is frequently encountered in daily clinical practice, and apparently during the acute phase of stroke about half of patients experience dysphagia. Since dysphagia affects ADL, QOL, and prognosis of the patients with stroke, it is of primary importance to find methods on how to handle dysphagia.

At present, the central pattern generator (CPG), which is located in the brainstem, is considered to be the swallowing center. The CPG consists of the solitary nucleus and the reticular formation and receives information from both hemispheres of the cerebral cortex. Neural input from the cerebral cortex that is transmitted to the CPG is conveyed via, e.g., the trigeminal nerve nucleus, facial nucleus, ambiguous nucleus, hypoglossal nucleus, and dorsal nucleus of the vagus nerve to swallowing-related muscle groups (Fig. 4.1). The CPG also receives input from peripheral receptors that are located in the oral cavity and pharynx via cranial nerves such as the trigeminal nerve, glossopharyngeal nerve, and vagus nerve.

In recent years, it has been increasingly emphasized that the smooth control of swallowing movements is not only regulated by the brainstem but also by the cerebral cortex. Allegedly the primary motor area, sensory area, insular cortex, and cingulate gyrus are important swallowing-related areas of the cerebral cortex. In most cases of dysphagia that are caused by supratentorial lesions, these lesions occur bilaterally. However, it is known that even if supratentorial lesions occur unilaterally approximately 30 % of patients develop dysphagia, and that in most of these patients dysphagia resolves within approximately 1 month. Therefore, it is

M. Abo, W. Kakuda, *Rehabilitation with rTMS*,
DOI 10.1007/978-3-319-20982-1_4

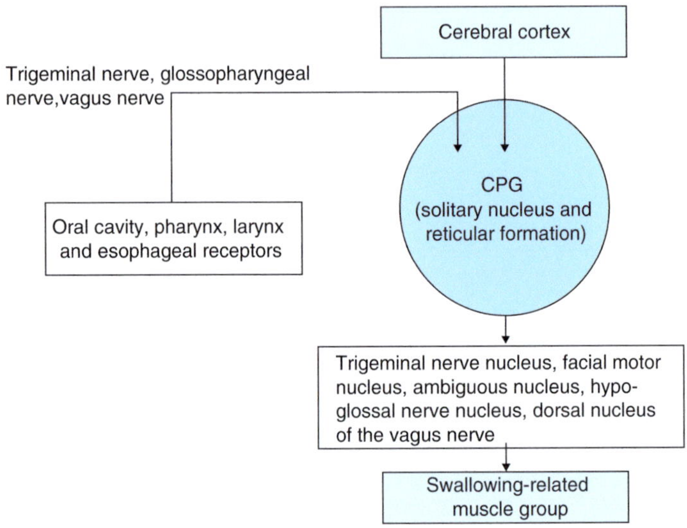

Fig. 4.1 Swallowing center. The swallowing center (CPG) is located in the brainstem. It is controlled by both hemispheres of the cortex, and also receives input from peripheral receptors

believed that in such cases the nonlesional hemisphere compensates for the affected hemisphere, and that this results in functional recovery.

It has been found that the stimulation of swallowing-related muscles by use of TMS (Fig. 4.2) results in the constriction caused by both hemispheres, which showed that swallowing-related muscles are controlled by both hemispheres. Moreover, although there are slight individual differences with respect to whether the right or left hemisphere is more dominant in terms of the control of swallowing, from our experience we have the impression that dominance of the right hemisphere is slightly more frequent. In cases where dysphagia is caused by unilateral lesions, there is a possibility that dysphagia results from damage to the originally dominant side.

B. Dysphagia Rehabilitation Methods

The following are three dysphagia rehabilitation methods that have been confirmed to be effective in comparative studies.

1) Head Raising Exercises

Head raising exercises are performed to strengthen the suprahyoid muscle group, improve movement of the hyoid bone and larynx, and reduce pharyngeal residues and aspiration [1].

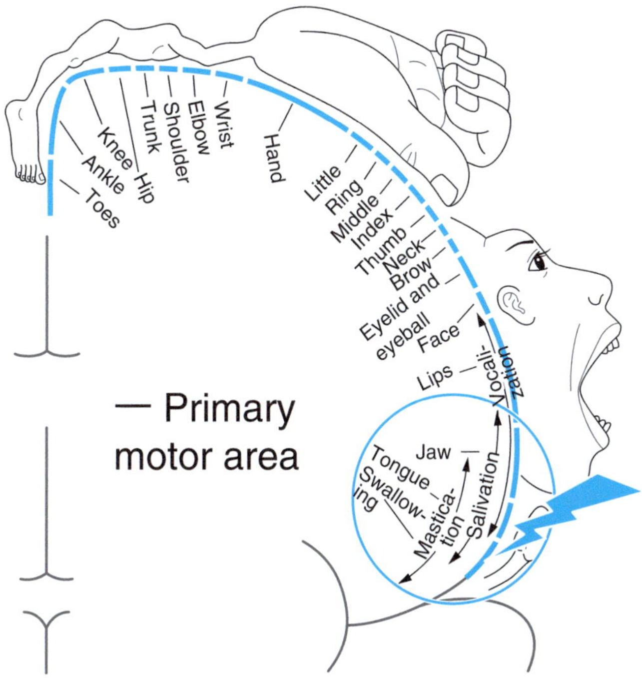

Fig. 4.2 Location of swallowing-related muscles in the primary motor cortex. As shown in Penfield's homunculus, all regions that represent swallowing-related muscles are located slightly below the lateral surface of the frontal lobe

2) McNeill Dysphagia Therapy Program

The McNeill dysphagia therapy program (MDTP) is a program in which foods of various consistency are to be swallowed for enhancing swallowing coordination. This program is characterized by combining single swallow strategies (to swallow foods or liquids in one attempt through strong swallowing) with remaining functions of the patient, and gradually food with a consistency that is increasingly difficult to swallow is given. When performing MDTP in patients with chronic dysphagia once daily for 1 hour over a period of 3 weeks, a significant improvement in findings on videofluoroscopic examination of swallowing was observed, and it was reported that this effect still was maintained 3 months later [2].

3) Electrical Stimulation of the Neck

Electrical stimulation of the neck is a method through which swallowing function is improved by electrical stimulation of the neck. This method has been reported to be useful [3], but there is no consensus on stimulation parameters and stimulation sites.

2 Idea Underlying the Application of rTMS in Combination with Dysphagia Rehabilitation

A. Previous Reports on the Application of rTMS

As of December 2012, when searching on MEDLINE the keywords "stroke, dysphagia, repetitive transcranial magnetic stimulation" we found 18 articles, and when searching the keywords "brain injury, dysphagia, repetitive transcranial magnetic stimulation" we found 5 articles. Among these were six research papers that actually examined the beneficial effects of rTMS on swallowing function in patients with poststroke dysphagia, which are shown in Table 4.1.

Khedr et al. [4] reported that swallowing function improved in the patients with supratentorial stroke when applying 3-Hz (120 %) high-frequency rTMS to the esophageal region of lesional primary motor area once daily over a period of 5 days. On the other hand, Verin et al. [5] reported that the swallowing reaction time, pharyngeal residue score, and aspiration score improved in the patients with supratentorial stroke when applying 1-Hz (120 %) low-frequency rTMS once daily for 20 minutes over a period of 5 days to the region of the nonlesional primary motor area that represents the laryngeal elevator muscle group. Moreover, Kim et al. [6] reported that when treating supratentorial stroke patients within 3 months after onset, the dysphagia scale as well as aspiration and laryngeal penetration improved more by low-frequency rTMS to the nonlesional hemisphere than by high-frequency rTMS to the lesional hemisphere. Besides, Michou et al. [7] reported that pharyngeal transit time, aspiration, and laryngeal penetration improved after performing paired-associative stimulation (PAS) by peripheral electrical stimulation and rTMS to the nonlesional primary motor area of patients with poststroke dysphagia. Furthermore, Park et al. [8] reported that in a double-blind RCT the dysphagia scale, aspiration, and laryngeal penetration significantly improved when applying 5-Hz (90 %) rTMS once daily for 20 minutes over a period of 2 weeks to the nonlesional pharyngeal motor area.

These reports are mainly on interventions that were performed in patients with supratentorial lesions; however, patients who had a subtentorial stroke, e.g., in the brainstem are actually those who suffer the most from dysphagia. Khedr et al. [9] reported that in patients with subtentorial stroke involving the brainstem and medulla oblongata, etc. the dysphagia scale significantly improved compared to the sham stimulation group (factitious stimulation) when performing 3-Hz (130 %) high-frequency stimulation once daily for 5 days to the esophageal region of primary motor area in both hemispheres (Fig. 4.3).

In a report on stimulation frequency and plasticity [10], MEP obtained after stimulation of the pharyngeal motor area at 1 Hz, 5 Hz, and 10 Hz were compared, and it was found that the largest MEPs were obtained after stimulation at 5 Hz (Fig. 4.4). Moreover, there is a report in which alterations in the MEPs of pharynx muscles were measured when applying rTMS not only to the cerebrum but also to the cerebellum [11], Based on these results it was considered that the cerebellum is involved in the regulation of swallowing process, and it was suggested that rTMS of the cerebellum might have an impact

Table 4.1 Research papers that examined the beneficial effects of rTMS on swallowing function

Name of author	Number of patients	Time from stroke onset	Stimulation sites	Stimulation methods	Clinical effects
Khedr EM, et al. (Acta Neurol Scand 2009)	26 stroke (unilateral cerebral lesion)	5–10 days	Lesional primary motor area	3 Hz (120 %)	Improved dysphagia score
Verin E, et al. (Dysphagia 2009)	7 stroke (2 cerebellar lesion)	11–132 months	Non-lesional primary motor area	1 Hz (120 %)	Improved swallowing response time, pharyngeal residue and aspiration score
Khedr EM, et al. (J Neurol Neurosurg Psychiatry 2010)	22 brainstem or medullary infarction	Within 3 months	Both primary motor cortices	3 Hz (130 %)	Improved grade of dysphagia
Kim L, et al. (Ann Rehabil Med 2011)	2 brain injury, 28 stroke (unilateral cerebral lesion)	Within 3 months	Lesional or non-lesional primary motor area	1 Hz or 5 Hz 100 %	Improved dysphagia scale, aspiration and laryngeal penetration at 1 Hz
Michou E, et al. (Gastroenterology 2012)	6 stroke (unilateral cerebral lesion)	6 months or longer (mean 38.8 weeks)	Non-lesional primary motor area	PAS	Improved pharynx transit time, aspiration and laryngeal penetration
Park JW, et al. (Neurogastroenterol Motil 2012)	18 stroke (unilateral cerebral lesion)	1–3 months	Non-lesional primary motor area x	5 Hz (90 %)	Improved dysphagia scale, aspiration and laryngeal penetration

on swallowing function. Moreover, in each study different methods were used for determining the stimulation site. In previous reports on rTMS for the treatment of dysphagia, the stimulation site was mostly determined by measuring MEP of the laryngeal elevator muscle group by use of a surface electromyogram of the neck or by measuring MEP of the laryngopharynx and esophagus by use of catheter electrodes (Fig. 4.5).

Even though all these treatment methods are termed rTMS for the treatment of poststroke dysphagia, as shown in Table 4.1, there exist various stimulation modalities, and also the stimulation method that we use at our facility is the result of continuous trial and error. At first, we were primarily concerned about the safety of the

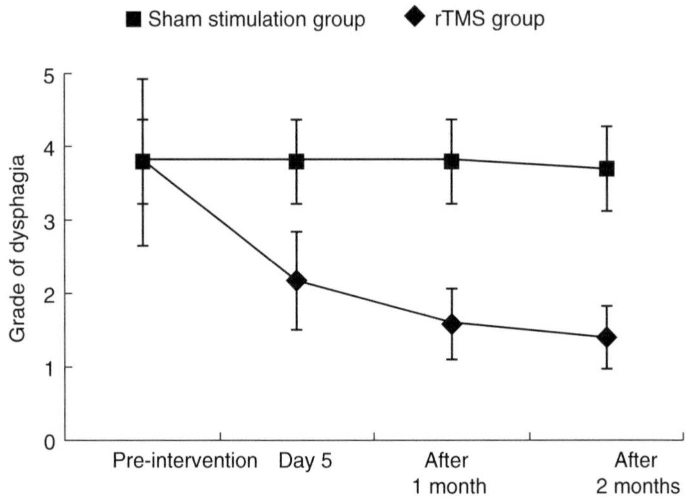

Fig. 4.3 Efficacy of bilateral magnetic stimulation. The dysphagia scale improved significantly more in the rTMS (3 Hz) group than in the sham stimulation group [7]

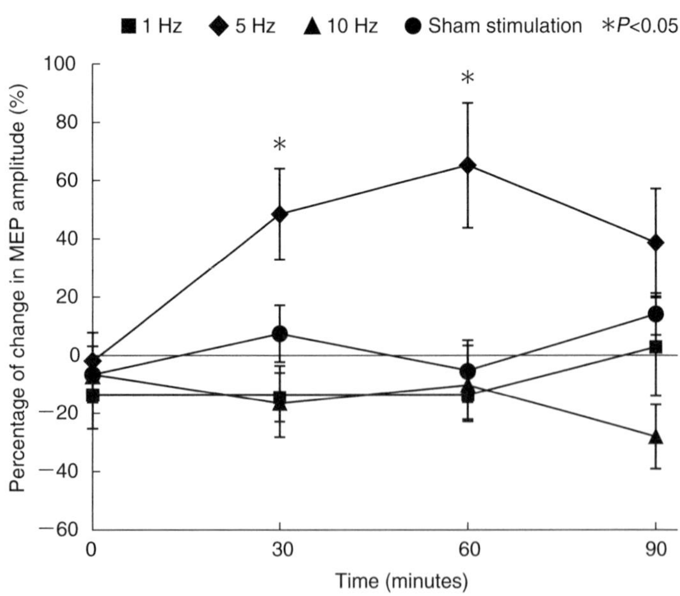

Fig. 4.4 Percentage of change in MEP amplitude by frequency. The greatest percentage of change in MEP amplitude (%) was obtained after stimulation at 5 Hz (Adapted from Ref. [10])

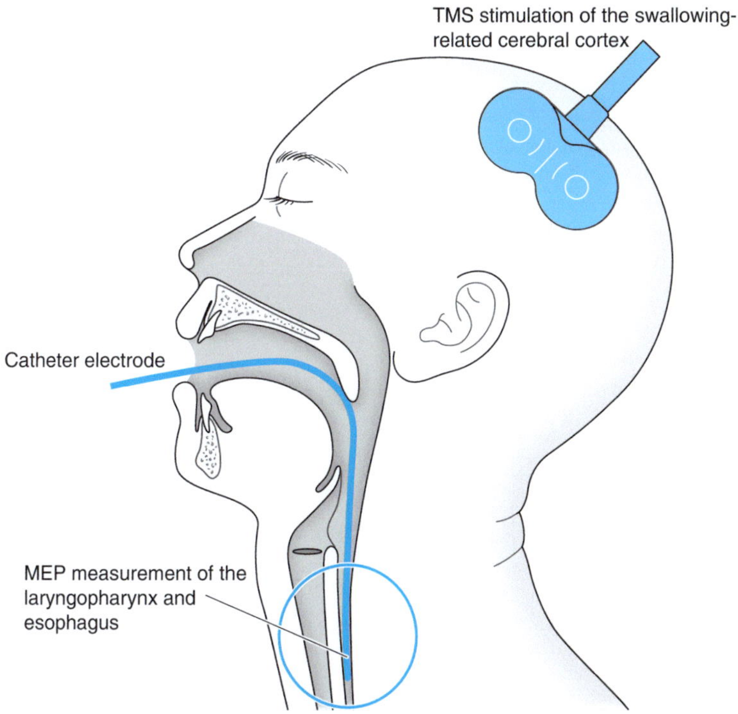

Fig. 4.5 Determination of the stimulation site by use of catheter electrodes. By use of a catheter that is inserted orally, MEPs of the laryngopharynx and esophagus are measured to determine the application sites of rTMS

patient and performed stimulation of the nonlesional hemisphere at 1 Hz. However, since there is only little lateralization in swallowing function because it is controlled by both hemispheres, and long-term dysphagia resulting from unilateral lesions is rare, at present we mostly use a bilateral rTMS (3–5 Hz) treatment protocol.

As described in the report in which bilateral stimulation was performed, the biggest advantage of this method is that one does not have to give too much thought to right or left laterality, and thus does not have to be concerned about the site of the lesion. Moreover, for increasing the plasticity of the pharyngeal region of primary motor area, we determine the stimulation site by measuring the MEP of pharyngeal muscles by use of catheter electrodes.

B. Eligibility Criteria for rTMS Treatment

Below are shown the eligibility criteria of rTMS for the treatment of poststroke dysphagia that are used at our hospital; however, they are only provisional (Table 4.2). Criterion 2 refers to patients in whom the use of rTMS is

Table 4.2 Eligibility criteria for rTMS for the treatment of poststroke dysphagia

1.	Presents with dysphagia caused by stroke (cerebral infarction, brain hemorrhage, or subarachnoid hemorrhage)
2.	No intracranial metal objects (e.g. a clip), or implanted cardiac pacemaker
3.	No recent history of convulsions at least within one year preceding the intervention (no abnormalities on electroencephalographic examination)
4.	No patient with severe dysphagia who constantly aspires saliva
5.	No patient with mild dysphagia, in whom the oral intake of a regular diet is possible
6.	Favorable general condition (no severe complications such as impaired consciousness, fever, or severe cardiac disease)
7.	Is not on dialysis
8.	No mental illness such as depression
9.	Underwent no tracheotomy, does not require aspiration, and also good respiratory status
10.	No recent history of pneumonia within three months preceding the intervention
11.	Can remain in a seated position for at least two hours, and does not require much assistance for daily living
12.	No significant cognitive impairment
13.	Is willing to undergo rehabilitation
14.	The age between 20 and 80 years

As of December, 2012

contraindicated, and criterion 3 was set up for excluding patients with epilepsy. Criterion 4 and 5 were set up for excluding patients with very severe or mild dysphagia, because from our experience in these patients rTMS is not very effective. Criteria 6 to 13 were set up for ensuring that the patient is in a condition that enables to perform intensive rehabilitation. Moreover, considering the patient's ability to give consent, we set up an age limit as can be seen in criterion 14 (we are planning to extend this age limit in the future).

C. Performing rTMS in Combination with Intensive Dysphagia Rehabilitation

Since the effects obtained by rTMS alone usually only last for a short period, long-term improvement requires dysphagia rehabilitation. Therefore, the patient is hospitalized for 1 to 2 weeks for performing rTMS and intensive dysphagia rehabilitation. Our treatment protocol is designed for rTMS that focuses on the pharyngeal phase of dysphagia, and therefore we consider it useful to combine this treatment with dysphagia rehabilitation for the pharyngeal phase of dysphagia. Specifically, we think that, e.g., the exercise for elevating the dorsum of the tongue, the tongue-hold-swallow exercise, mouth opening exercise [12], head raising exercise, effortful swallowing exercise (Table 4.3), and MDTP may be useful.

Table 4.3 Dysphagia rehabilitation in combination with rTMS treatment

Dorsum of tongue raising exercise	The dorsum of the tongue is depressed e.g. with a tongue depressor, and the patient is asked to resist the applied pressure by lifting his tongue, and to hold this position for a few seconds. This exercise is expected to enhance pharyngeal pressure
Tongue-hold-swallow exercise	The patient is asked to project the tongue tip forward, and to swallow saliva while keeping the tongue on his front teeth. This exercise is expected to enhance pharyngeal contraction force
Mouth opening exercise	The patient is asked to open his/her mouth as wide as possible and to hold this position for a few seconds. Then this exercise is repeated several times. This exercise is expected to increase the dilation rate of the esophageal orifice, and to improve the pharyngeal transit time
Head raising exercise	The patient is in a supine position and raises only his/her head until he/she can see his/her toe. The duration and repetition of this movement are adjusted as appropriate. Promotes bolus transit into the esophageal entrance, and reduces pharyngeal residues
Effortful swallowing exercise	The patients is asked to swallow as if squeezing something by putting force into the swallowing muscle group while pressing the tongue against the palate. Strengthens backward movement of the tongue root, and reduces pharyngeal residues

3 Protocol of rTMS in Combination with Intensive Dysphagia Rehabilitation

A. Treatment Overview

The hospitalization schedule for rTMS for the treatment of poststroke dysphagia at our department is shown in Table 4.4. In detail rTMS is applied twice daily in the morning and evening (except for the day of hospitalization/discharge and Sundays) to the pharyngeal motor cortex in both hemispheres for 10 seconds alternatively to the left and right hemisphere at 3–5 Hz (90–130 %), followed by a rest of 20 seconds, and this cycle is repeated 20 times (in total 10 minutes) (Table 4.5). Hereafter, indirect-swallowing exercises are performed for 20 minutes under the guidance of a speech therapist. Moreover, patients who are able to conduct self-exercise do additional indirect-swallowing exercises by themselves.

Usually patients are hospitalized for 6 days; they are admitted on Monday and discharged on Saturday. rTMS is conducted for 6 consecutive days, except on Sundays, and if the length of hospitalization is not limited it can be extended up to 15 days. Moreover, at the time of admission stimulation site and the intensity of stimulation are determined, and swallowing function is evaluated, and at the time of discharge swallowing function is re-evaluated.

By use of a catheter electrode (we mostly use catheter electrodes from Gaeltec Ltd.) the site at which the largest MEPs are elicited in pharyngeal muscles is

Table 4.4 An example of the hospitalization schedule used when performing rTMS for the treatment of dysphagia[a]

	Mon	Tue to Fri	Sat
Morning	Evaluation at admission	rTMS (10 minutes)	
		Dysphagia rehabilitation (20 minutes)	
Afternoon	rTMS (10 minutes)		Evaluation at discharge
	Dysphagia rehabilitation (20 minutes)		

[a]If hospitalized on Monday
As of December, 2012

Table 4.5 An example of rTMS performed for the treatment of dysphagia

Coil used	Figure-8 coil
Stimulation site	Both hemispheres (pharyngeal region of primary motor area)
Intensity	90–130 % of motor threshold
Frequency	3–5 Hz
Duration	1 session lasting 10 minutes, once or twice daily
Number of days of hospitalization	Usually 6 days (maximum 15 days)

As of December, 2012

determined and set as stimulation site on the cerebrum. First, in the imaging room of our department, MEPs are measured after having confirmed the position of the catheter electrodes on the pharynx (Fig. 4.6). Determination of the stimulation site when using catheter electrodes is a reliable method; however, it is quite cumbersome and complicated. Therefore in difficult cases, it is also possible to measure instead the MEPs that are elicited in the suprahyoid muscle group, which is also easier. For measuring the MEPs that are elicited in the suprahyoid muscle group, the electrodes should be placed between the hyoid bone and the mentum (Fig. 4.7). Besides, it is also conceivable that the stimulation site can be determined by visually confirming the movement of pharyngeal muscles resulting from TMS by videoendoscopic examination of swallowing.

B. Evaluation of Swallowing Function

At our department, before and after performing rTMS change in swallowing function is evaluated by use of a highly reliable evaluation method such as those described below.

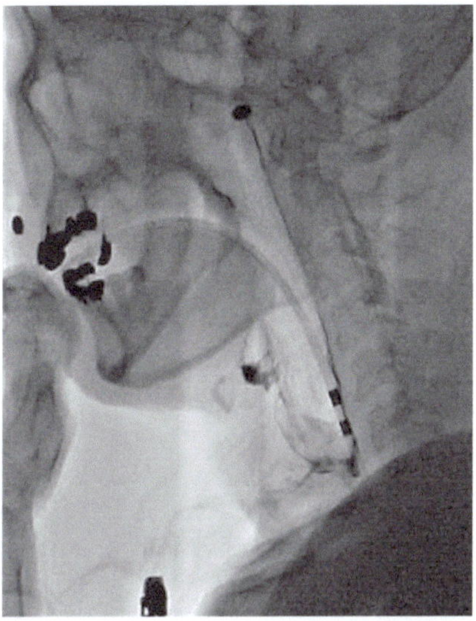

Fig. 4.6 Example showing the insertion of a catheter electrode. At our department the position of the catheter is checked by imaging

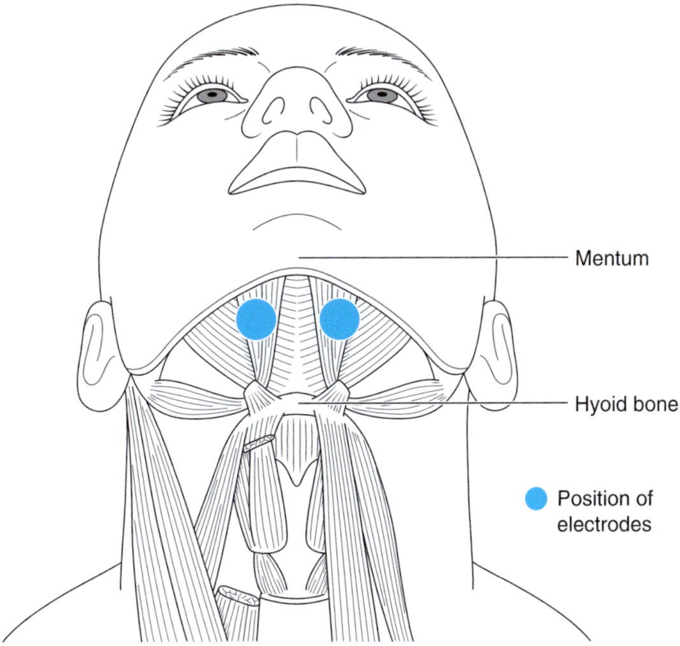

Fig. 4.7 Laryngeal elevator muscle group and position of electrodes. The stimulation site can also be determined by placing an electrode between the hyoid bone and the mentum

1) Repetitive Saliva Swallowing Test

There are some reports on that the number of voluntary swallowing increased by rTMS for the treatment of dysphagia. With the repetitive saliva swallowing test (RSST) [13], the number of times that the patient is able to swallow saliva within 30 seconds is checked, and the number of times that the patient is able to swallow saliva within 60 seconds is recorded in combination with inspection, palpation, and auscultation.

2) Mann Assessment of Swallowing Ability (MASA)

This test is widely used worldwide. It consists of 24 examination items and a 200-point grading scale, and is used for the quantitative assessment of the severity of poststroke dysphagia. The higher the score, the better are the swallowing functions of the patient. This test is also used, for instance, for the assessment of quantitative effect in the studies of interventions for dysphagia. Also its revised version, MMASA [14], which consists of 12 examination items and a 100-point grading scale, has been reported to be reliable and valid for assessing poststroke dysphagia.

3) Functional Oral Intake Scale (FOIS)

With this scale the actual oral intake of the patient is assessed based on seven levels [15]. The more difficult the food or liquid items the patient is able to take in orally, the higher the score. Moreover, another scale that is similar to the FOIS scale is the food intake LEVEL scale (FILS) [16]. FILS is frequently used in Japan and is made up of 10 levels of oral intake ability.

4) Clinical Dysphagia Scale (CDS)

This is a 100-point grading scale that is made up of 8 examination items, namely, site of lesion, tracheotomy, aspiration, lip sealing, chewing and mastication, tongue protrusion, laryngeal elevation, and reflex coughing. The higher the score, the more severe the degree of dysphagia (Table 4.6) [17].

5) Videofluoroscopic Dysphagia Scale (VDS)

This is a 100-point grading scale that is made up of 14 examination items based on which findings on videofluoroscopy of swallowing are evaluated, and it has been reported to be used, e.g., for poststroke dysphagia prognosis prediction (Table 4.7) [18]. This scale is also frequently used for assessing the effect in studies on intervention for dysphagia.

Table 4.6 Clinical dysphagia scale (CDS)

Outcome measures		Scores	Outcome measures		Scores
Location	Non-stem lesion	0	Tongue protrusion	Intact	0
	Stem lesion	5		Inadequate	4
Tracheotomy	No	0		None	8
	Yes	25	Laryngeal elevation	Intact	0
Aspiration	No	0		Inadequate	5
	Yes	10		None	10
Lip sealing	Intact	0	Reflex coughing	No	0
	Inadequate	2		Yes	30
	None	4			
Chewing and mastification	Intact	0			
	Inadequate	4			
	None	8	Total		/100

Reference [17]

Table 4.7 Videofluoroscopic dysphagia scale (VDS)

Outcome measures		Score	Outcome measures		Score
Lip closure	Intact	0	Triggering of pharyngeal swallow	Normal	0
	Inadequate	2		Delayed	4.5
	None	4	Vallecular residue	None	0
Bolus formation	Intact	0		<10 %	2
	Inadequate	3		10–50 %	4
	None	6		>50 %	6
Mastification	Intact	0	Laryngeal elevation	Normal	0
	Inadequate	4		Impaired	0
	None	8	Pyriform sinus residue	None	0
Apraxia	None	0		<10 %	4.5
	Mild	1.5		10–50 %	9
	Moderate	3		>50 %	13.5
	Severe	4.5	Coating of the pharyngeal wall	No	0
Tongue-to-palate contact	Intact	0		Yes	9
	Inadequate	5	Pharynx transit time	≦1.0 s	0
	None	10		>1.0 s	6
Premature bolus loss	None	0	Aspiration	None	0
	<19 %	1.5		Supraglottic penetration	6
	10–50 %	3			
	>50 %	4.5		Subglottic penetration	12
Oral transit time	≦1.5 s	0			
	>1.5 s	3	Total		/100

Reference [18]

6) Penetration-Aspiration Scale (P-A Scale)

This is an 8-point grading scale with which the severity of laryngeal penetration and aspiration can be assessed, and it is generally evaluated by using videofluoroscopy of swallowing [19]. The higher the score, the more severe the degree of laryngeal penetration and aspiration.

7) Laryngeal Elevation Delay Time (LEDT)

This is a swallowing examination that is performed by use of contrast material, and the results are expressed as the laryngeal elevation delay time at which maximum laryngeal elevation occurs after the contrast material reaches the esophageal entrance. It has been reported that with this method the LEDT can easily be quantitatively determined and that effects on the site of cerebral infarction are reflected with high sensitivity [20].

8) Swallowing Quality of Life (SWAL-QOL)

This is a rating scale using a dysphagia-specific self-completed QOL questionnaire, in which 44 questions on 11 areas related to swallowing are to be answered in 4–6 grades and then are assessed by a rating scale [21]. The results of each subscale are scored using a 100-point grading scale, and then expressed in a multidimensional profile. The higher the score, the higher the QOL (Table 4.8) [22]. A Japanese version has also been developed that is used together with SWAL-CARE, which is a questionnaire on the patient's satisfaction with the explanations he or she was provided regarding feeding methods and treatment and the patient's satisfaction with the medical staff [22].

4 Treatment Outcomes in Our Department

In this section we present the outcomes of rTMS for the treatment of poststroke dysphagia at our department.

A. Study Patients

We treated four patients who developed dysphagia resulting from cerebral infarction, three women and one man (Table 4.9). Age at the time of intervention ranged from 56 to 80 years old, and the time to treatment initiation from the onset of cerebral infarction ranged from 6 to 37 months. The subtype and location of cerebral infarction were diagnosed within 30 days before the start of treatment by use of

MRI. Two patients were diagnosed with bilateral cerebral infarction, one with bilateral cerebellar infarction, and one with left medullar infarction. Levels of oral food intake in these patients ranged widely, namely, from level 1 to 6 out of 7, when assessed by use of the FOIS scale.

B. Method

1) Treatment Schedule

As described above, the patients were hospitalized and underwent treatment for 6 days. In the afternoon of the day of hospitalization rTMS was performed for 10 minutes, followed by 20 minutes of one-to-one dysphagia rehabilitation. Hereafter,

Table 4.8 SWAL-QOL subscale[a]

1. Burden (Burd)
2. Eating duration (Eatdur)
3. Eating desire (Eatdes)
4. Food selection (Food)
5. Communication (Com)
6. Fear (Fear)
7. Mental health (MH)
8. Social function (Social)
9. Sleep (Sleep)
10. Fatigue (Fatig)

[a]Items included in the outcome profile

Reference [22]

Table 4.9 Clinical characteristics of studied patients

No	Age at intervention (years)	Gender	Time between onset and intervention	Site of stroke lesion	NIHSS[a]	FIM[b]
Patient 1	80	Female	24 months	Both cerebral hemispheres	5	92
Patient 2	67	Male	7 months	Left medulla oblongata	4	88
Patient 3	69	Female	6 months	Both cerebral hemispheres	5	95
Patient 4	56	Female	37 months	Both cerebellar hemispheres	5	96

[a]NIHSS (national institute of health stroke scale)

[b]FIM (functional independence measure)

this double treatment session was conducted twice daily in the morning and afternoon, on consecutive days.

2) rTMS Treatment Protocol

rTMS was performed by use of MagPro R30 and a figure-8 coil (both manufactured by MagVenture). Stimulation was performed at 3 Hz for 10 seconds (1 cycle) at intervals of 30 seconds, alternatively to the left and right primary motor cortex, and this cycle was repeated 20 times. The stimulation site was set as the location where the largest MEPs were measured for the pharyngeal muscle group by use of a catheter electrode, and the stimulation intensity was set at 130 % of the resting motor threshold derived from both the right and left abductor pollicis brevis.

3) Dysphagia Rehabilitation Program

After rTMS indirect-swallowing exercises, which were a combination of tongue movements, head raising and effortful swallowing exercises were performed in one-on-one training with a speech therapist for approximately 20 minutes, twice daily.

(i) Tongue movements included exercises such as protruding out the tongue and then drawing it back, or pressing the dorsum of the tongue against a finger, and were to be performed four to five times each, only to the extent possible without causing pain.
(ii) During the head raising exercise the patients were in a supine position with their shoulders attached to the floor, and should raise only their head until they could see their toe, followed by three-time repetition of "holding this position for one minute, followed a one minute rest." If it was difficult for a patient to raise his or her head continuously for 1 minute, the duration of this exercise was set at 50 % of the maximum possible time that the patient was able to continuously raise his/her head.
(iii) For the effortful swallowing exercise, patients were asked to press their tongue as strongly as possible against the palate "if possible for 30 seconds, followed by a rest of 30 seconds," and this was repeated two to three times.

If these exercises caused pain or fatigue on the following day, exercises were adjusted to the extent that they did not cause pain or fatigue.

4) Evaluation of Swallowing Function

Swallowing function was evaluated on the day of admission and discharge by videofluoroscopy examination of swallowing. Contrast medium was to be swallowed three times, and swallowing was evaluated based on the worst scores on the P-A scale and for LEDT. Moreover, also evaluation based on MMASA, RSST, and FOIS was performed.

C. Result

This 6-day combination treatment was completed without observing, e.g., convulsions, an aggravation of neurological symptoms, or pneumonia. Endoscopic observation of the pharynx during rTMS revealed the occurrence of swallowing-like movements. As for changes in swallowing function, a tendency of improved MMASA scores and LEDT was observed. Scores on the P-A scale, RSST, and FOIS were also unchanged or showed a trend of improvement (Table 4.10), and in no patient an aggravation of dysphagia was observed. Moreover, an improvement in the ability of oral intake and a reduction in repeated choking were observed when patients were actually taking their meals.

D. Discussion

No adverse events were observed in any of the patients in whom we carried out this treatment protocol, and therefore we believe that this treatment method is safe and highly feasible. Swallowing function is thought to be controlled bilaterally, but hemispheric dominance has also been reported [23]. However, in clinical practice, it is sometimes difficult to identify which is the dominant side, and therefore methods such as bilateral rTMS, which can be performed without having to be concerned about laterality, are highly versatile. In this study, in all patients an improvement in the triggering speed to swallowing reflex was observed.

Compared with conventional rehabilitation, the methods that we used in this treatment protocol do not require the direct use of food and therefore possibly are also safe in patients who have difficulty taking in food orally. Moreover, possibly also treatment goals that we could not sufficiently investigate in this study such as improved pharyngeal contraction force, prevention of aspiration pneumonia by reducing nocturnal saliva aspiration, and depending on the stimulation site, increased tongue pressure, improved coordination of mastication, and improved gastroesophageal reflux can be achieved in the future. Furthermore, in future studies it needs to be investigated for which subtypes or severity of stroke this treatment is effective and the timing of treatment initiation from onset. We also believe that by elucidating which symptoms of dysphagia can be improved, a more appropriate rehabilitation program can be devised.

5 Future Challenges

Attempts to use rTMS for the treatment of poststroke dysphagia have just begun, and further investigation needs to be conducted in the future. We conclude this chapter by giving an overview of the main items that require further investigation.

Table 4.10 Changes in the evaluation of swallowing function resulting from treatment

Assessment method	Patient 1		Patient 2		Patient 3		Patient 4	
	Pre-treatment	Post-treatment	Pre-treatment	Post-treatment	Pre-treatment	Post-treatment	Pre-treatment	Post-treatment
MMASA[a]	87	90	43	55	78	82	73	69
P-A scale[b]	4	1	5	2	5	2	3	3
LEDT (seconds)[c]	0.12	0.08	0.52	0.08	3.96	0.12	0.36	0.12
RSST[d]	1	2	1	1	1	2	0	0
FOIS[e]	5	6	1	2	2	3	6	6

[a]MMASA (modified Mann assessment of swallowing ability)
[b]P-A scale (penetration-aspiration scale)
[c]LEDT (laryngeal elevation delay time)
[d]RSST (repetitive saliva swallowing test)
[e]FOIS (functional oral intake scale)

1) Indications

We have the impression that when treating poststroke dysphagia by use of rTMS there are both responders who benefit from treatment and nonresponders who do not. It would be helpful if it were possible to distinguish between responders and nonresponders prior to intervention; however, currently this is not possible.

2) Treatment Protocol

In the future, detailed further investigation is required with regard to the stimulation site, intensity, frequency, details on rehabilitation exercises that should be conducted in combination with rTMS, as well as on the optimal timing of rTMS application after onset of stroke. There is also a possibility that in some cases, depending on the characteristics of the patient, this stimulation method needs to be applied in a slightly different manner.

3) Long-Term Effects

The duration of the effects that are achieved by rTMS require further investigation. At present, the long-term benefits of rTMS in patients with dysphagia have yet to be studied sufficiently. However, in patients who could be followed up after discharge, the effects of rTMS appeared to have persisted.

4) Beneficial Effects

The kinds of improvements that can be achieved by use of rTMS require further investigation. We think that it is necessary to assess multiple aspects with regard to the effects of rTMS in patients with dysphagia, such as measuring swallowing pressure before and after intervention.

References

1. Crary MA, Carnaby GD, LaGorio LA, et al. Functional and physiological outcomes from an exercise-based dysphagia therapy; a pilot investigation of the McNeill Dysphagia Therapy Program. Arch Phys Med Rehabil. 2012;93:1173–8.
2. Shaker R, Easterling C, Kern M, et al. Rehabilitation of swallowing by exercise in tube-fed patients with pharyngeal dysphagia secondary to abnormal UES opening. Gastroenterology. 2002;122:1314–21.

3. Freed ML, Freed L, Chatburn RL, et al. Electrical stimulation for swallowing disorders caused by stroke. Respir Care. 2001;46:466–74.
4. Khedr EM, Abo-Elfetoh N, Rothwell J. Treatment of post-stroke dysphagia with repetitive transcranial magnetic stimulation. Acta Neurol Scand. 2009;119:155–61.
5. Verin E, Leroi A. Poststroke dysphagia rehabilitation by repetitive transcranial magnetic stimulation: a noncontrolled pilot study. Dysphagia. 2009;24:204–10.
6. Kim L, Chun MH, Kim BR, et al. Effect of repetitive transcranial magnetic stimulation on patients with brain injury and dysphagia. Ann Rehab Med. 2010;35:765–71.
7. Michou E, Mistry S, Jefferson S, et al. Targeting unlesioned pharyngeal motor cortex improves swallowing in healthy individuals and after dysphagic stroke. Gastroenterology. 2012;142:29–38.
8. Park JW, Oh JC, Lee JW, et al. The effect of 5Hz high-frequency rTMS over contralesional pharyngeal motor cortex in post-stroke oropharyngeal dysphagia; a randomized controlled study. Neurogastroenterol Motil. 2013;25:324–e250.
9. Khedr EM, Abo-Elfetoh N. Therapeutic role of rTMS on recovery of dysphagia in patients with lateral medullary syndrome and brainstem infarction. J Neurol Neurosurg Psychiatry. 2010;81:495–9.
10. Gow D, Rothwell J, Hobson A, et al. Induction of long-term plasticity in human swallowing motor cortex following repetitive cortical stimulation. Clin Neurophysiol. 2004;115:1044–51.
11. Jayasekeran V, Rothwell J, Hamdy S. Non-invasive magnetic stimulation of the human cerebellum facilitates cortico-bulbar projections in the swallowing motor system. Neurogastroenterol Motil. 2011;23:831–e341.
12. Wada S, Tohara H, Iida T, et al. Jaw-opening exercise for insufficient opening of upper esophageal sphincter. Arch Phys Med Rehabil. 2012;93:1995–9.
13. Oguchi K, Saitoh E, Baba M, et al. The repetitive saliva swallowing test (RSST) as a screening test of functional dysphagia (2) validity of RSST. Jpn J Rehab Med. 2000;37:383–8. Japanese.
14. Antonios N, Carnaby-Mann G, Crary M, et al. Analysis of a physician tool for evaluating dysphagia on an inpatient stroke unit: the modified Mann Assessment of Swallowing Ability. J Stroke Cerebrovasc Dis. 2010;19:49–57.
15. Crary MA, Mann GDC, Groher ME. Initial psychometric assessment of a functional oral intake scale for dysphagia in stroke patients. Arch Phys Med Rehabil. 2005;86:1516–20.
16. Kunieda K, Ohno T, Fujishima I, et al. Reliability and validity of a tool to measure the severity of dysphagia: the food intake LEVEL scale. J Pain Symptom Manage 15 Nov 2012.
17. Chun SW, Lee SA, Jung IY, et al. Inter-rater agreement for the clinical dysphagia scale. Ann Rehab Med. 2011;35:470–6.
18. Han TR, Paik NJ, Park JW, et al. The prediction of persistent dysphagia beyond six months after stroke. Dysphagia. 2008;23:59–64.
19. Rosenbek JC, Robbins JA, Roecker EB, et al. A penetration-aspiration scale. Dysphagia. 1996;1:93–8.
20. Miyaji H, Umezaki T, Adachi K, et al. Videofluoroscopic assessment of pharyngeal stage delay reflects pathophysiology after brain infarction. Laryngoscope. 2012;122:2793–9.
21. McHorney CA, Robbins J, Lomax K, et al. The SWAL-QOL and SWAL-CARE outcomes tool for oropharyngeal dysphagia in adults: III. Documentation of reliability and validity. Dysphagia. 2002;17:97–114.
22. Wada M, Hoshino Y, Okudaira N, et al. QOL evaluation of patients with dysphagia — a comparative study of the application of a comprehensive QOL questionnaire (SF-36) and the trial use of disease-specific QOL questionnaires (SWAL-QOL, SWAL-CARE). Jpn J Dysphagia Rehab. 2003;7:109–16. Japanese.
23. Hamdy S, Aziz Q, Rothwell JC, et al. The cortical topography of human swallowing musculature in health and disease. Nat Med. 1966;2:1217–24.

Chapter 5
rTMS for Lower Limb Hemiparesis after Stroke

Whether patients with poststroke hemiparesis have a gait disturbance or not is closely related to a drop in ADL level and a deterioration in QOL.

According to Copenhagen Stroke Study [1], 50 % of patients with stroke are unable to walk independently at the time of onset, but 80 % may regain ambulatory ability through subsequent rehabilitation. Even if ambulatory ability has been regained, problems such as slowed walking speed, a right-left difference between lower limbs in taking a step forward, a right-left difference between lower limbs in muscle strength, spasticity in the paralyzed lower limb, and foot drop are common. In fact, many patients have some residual gait disturbances.

In recent years, the use of gait training devices such as Lokomat and Gait Trainer has drawn attention [2]. For example, body-weight supported treadmill training (BWSTT) is designed for patients with a gait disturbance induced by poststroke lower limb hemiparesis and involves the use of a harness to facilitate gait training on a treadmill while controlling the burden on the paralyzed lower limb. Unlike in cases of poststroke upper limb hemiparesis, however, there are very few reports of the successful application of noninvasive brain stimulation to poststroke lower limb hemiparesis.

Despite this, it may still be possible to use rTMS as a therapeutic intervention against a gait disturbance induced by poststroke lower limb hemiparesis, considering the neuromodulation effects of rTMS. We began attempting application of rTMS to gait disturbance induced by poststroke lower limb hemiparesis. We are already seeing some good signs.

This chapter is about our commitment to the therapeutic application of rTMS to a gait disturbance induced by poststroke lower limb hemiparesis.

M. Abo, W. Kakuda, *Rehabilitation with rTMS*,
DOI 10.1007/978-3-319-20982-1_5

1 Difference between Lower Limb Hemiparesis and Upper Limb Hemiparesis

At least two significant differences exist between poststroke lower and upper limb hemiparesis. First, there is a difference in localization between the lower and upper limb regions of the primary motor area. Known as Penfield's homunculus, the localization of sites in the primary motor area corresponding to each of the body parts is clear. The upper limb region in the primary motor area exists on the lateral surface of the frontal lobe that is located in a shallow area from the surface of the head. In contrast, the lower limb region of the primary motor area is located in the deep, namely, the medial frontal lobe, and areas for the left and right limbs are adjacent to each other (Fig. 5.1). The figure-8 coil used in the treatment of upper limb hemiparesis (p. 10) is considered to have its focus of stimulation at a relatively shallow area. With such a figure-8 coil, however, the magnetic stimulation may be insufficiently delivered to the lower limb region of the primary motor area.

The other difference involves the importance of nerve fibers that derive from the ipsilateral hemisphere and do not cross to the opposite hemisphere. In a healthy

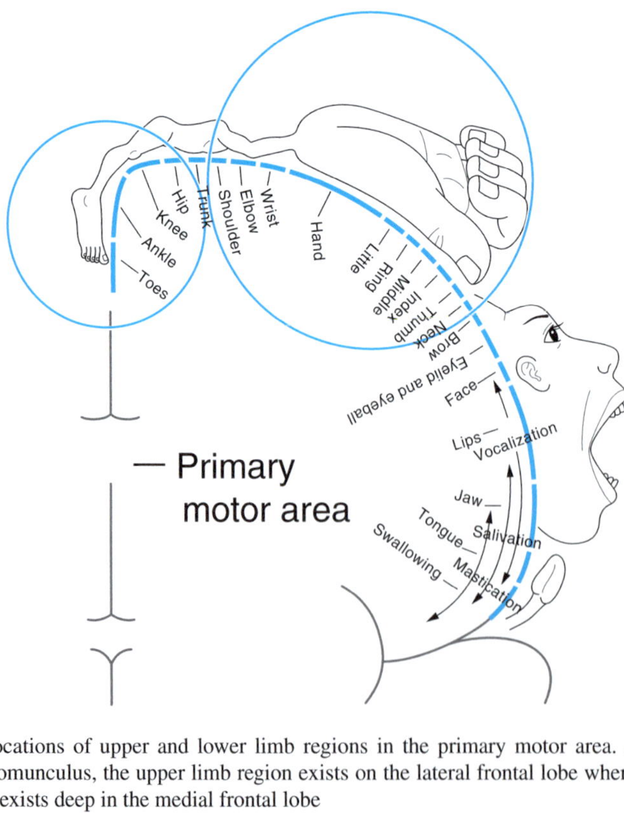

Fig. 5.1 Locations of upper and lower limb regions in the primary motor area. As shown by Penfield's homunculus, the upper limb region exists on the lateral surface frontal lobe whereas the lower limb region exists deep in the medial frontal lobe

person, most of the motor function in the upper limbs (probably 90 % or more) is governed by the contralateral hemisphere. In other words, the nerve fibers that derive from the contralateral hemisphere and cross through the pyramis medullae oblongatae are considered to govern most of the motor function of upper limbs. However, nerve fibers deriving from the contralateral hemisphere account for only 70–80 % of the motor function of lower limbs while the remaining 20–30 % is considered to be governed by the nerve fibers that derive from the ipsilateral hemisphere and do not cross to the opposite hemisphere (Fig. 5.2) [3, 4].

Some reports have confirmed and demonstrated the importance of the nerve fibers deriving from the ipsilateral hemisphere in the process of recovery from

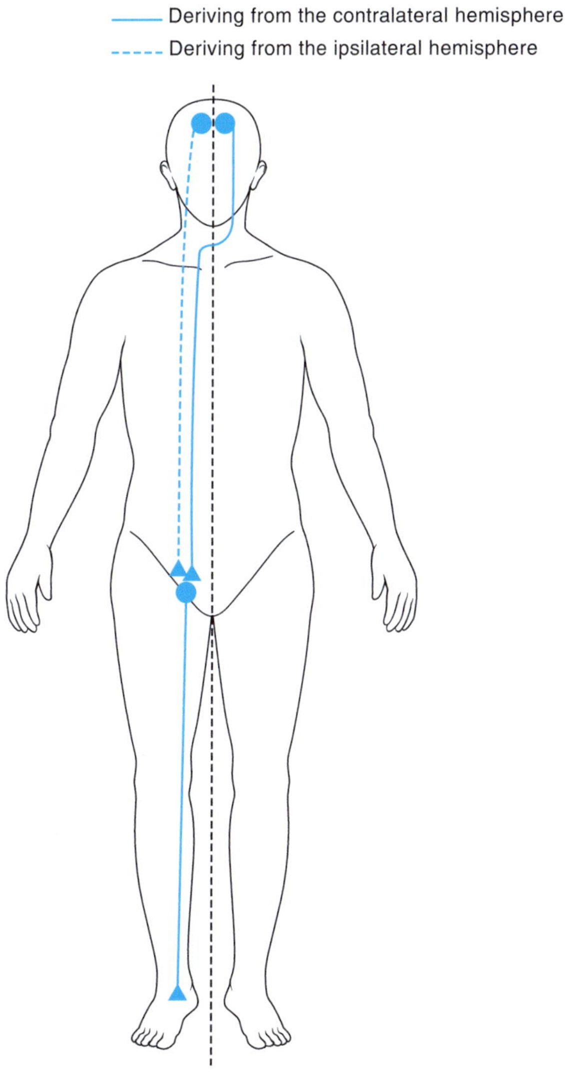

Fig. 5.2 Innervation of the motor function in the lower limbs. To some extent, the motor function in the lower limbs is also governed by the nerve fibers that derive from the ipsilateral hemisphere and do not cross to the opposite hemisphere

poststroke lower limb hemiparesis, with the use of nerve function images. Luft et al. [5] reported that poststroke patients whose gait function achieved remarkable improvement were accompanied by the activation of the primary motor area in the nonlesional hemisphere, which was confirmed by the functional MRI. Enzinger et al. [6] say the degree of activation of the bilateral primary motor area in the functional MRI correlates with the recovery of poststroke gait function. Similarly, Yen et al. [7] discuss the need for activating the bilateral hemisphere in the recovery of poststroke motor function in the lower limbs, based on the study using the TMS mapping.

Considering the differences between the upper limb and the lower limb motor system, it may be necessary to ensure that "the magnetic stimulation reaches the lower limb region of the primary motor area which is located in a deep area," provided that rTMS is to be therapeutically applied to poststroke lower limb hemiparesis. It may also be necessary to "activate the lower limb region of the unaffected primary motor area in addition to the lower limb region of the affected primary motor area."

In response to this, a double cone coil has been clinically applied in recent years. This is a set of two circular coils connected with each other at an angle ranging between 90 and 120 degrees. It is designed to have a deep focus of stimulation, namely, the point at which the magnetic stimulation concentrates (Fig. 5.3). The safety of the double cone coil in a human body has already been demonstrated. Using this coil is also reported to facilitate magnetic stimulation in the lower limb region of the primary motor area. According to Stokić et al. [8], using the double cone coil to give stimulation to a healthy person made it possible to record the MEP from the lower limb muscles such as tibialis anterior. Terao et al. [9] published a similar report.

Based on these findings, it is quite possible that the application of the double cone coil on the cranial median line, as shown in Fig. 5.4, could simultaneously stimulate the lower limb regions of the bilateral primary motor area.

Fig. 5.3 Double cone coil. This coil is designed to have a focus of stimulation in a deep position. The coil in the photo is Cool D-B80 (manufactured by MagVenture)

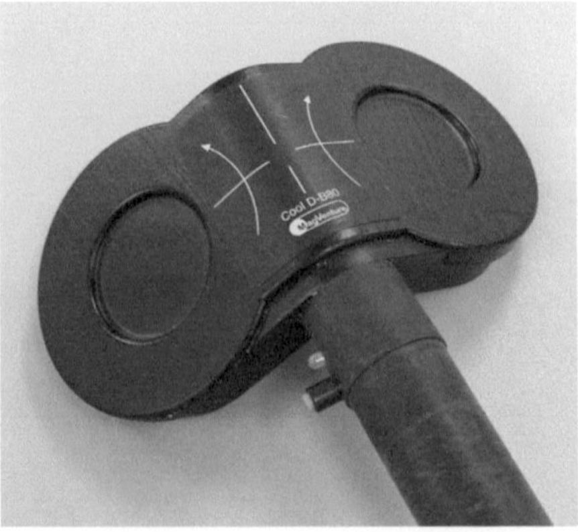

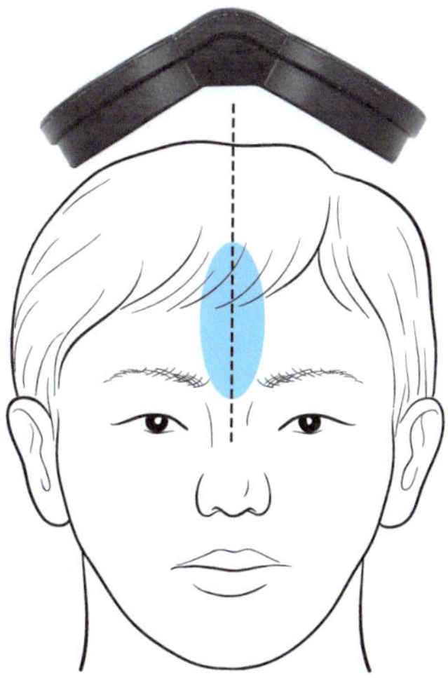

Fig. 5.4 Application of the double cone coil. Applying the coil on the cranial median line enables to simultaneously stimulate the lower limb regions of the primary motor area on both sides

2 Usefulness of High-Frequency rTMS with the Use of a Double Cone Coil

Based on the abovementioned view, we decided to conduct a crossover study to learn how the high-frequency rTMS on the lower limb region of the primary motor area on both sides of the cerebrum using a double cone coil influences the gait function of poststroke patients with lower limb hemiparesis. In other words, we sought to clarify the effects of high-frequency rTMS on gait functions by applying high-frequency rTMS using a double cone coil and sham stimulation on all patients and evaluating their gait function before and after each stimulation [10].

A. Patients

The study enrolled 18 patients with a gait disturbance and chronic poststroke hemiparesis. The eligibility criteria were set as shown in Table 5.1 in consideration of the guidelines of Wassermann [11] and similar. Table 5.2 shows the clinical background of the patients. The mean age of patients was 52.1 years old, and the mean time from onset to study enrollment was 52.8 months. The causal type of stroke was intracerebral bleeding in 13 patients and cerebral infarction in 5 patients.

B. Methods

The study was designed as a crossover study in which all patients receive both high-frequency rTMS and sham stimulation for 20 minutes each. In other words, half of the patients received the high-frequency rTMS and had an interval of at least 24 hours

Table 5.1 Eligibility criteria for indication of rTMS treatment for lower limb hemiparesis

1. Although an onset of stroke has induced a gait disturbance, the patient is capable of walking at least 10 meters by themselves without using a cane or a walking aid
2. The age between 30 and 70 at the time of the study
3. Time between the stroke onset and the study enrollment of more than 12 months
4. History of a single stroke only (neither recurrent nor bilateral)
5. No active systemic or mental illness requiring medical management
6. The patient has not received motor point block, botulinum toxin or other procedure for local treatment of lower limb spasms
7. The patient has no history of spasticity
8. No abnormality is recognizable in an electroencephalography
9. No abnormality is The patient has no contraindications specified in the Wassermann's guideline (intracranial metals, a cardiac pacemaker and pregnancy) in an electroencephalography

As of December 2012

Table 5.2 Clinical background of patients[a]

Age		52.1 ± 11.9 years old
Time from the onset of stroke		52.8 ± 30.7 months
Gender	Men	13 (72 %)
	Women	5 (28 %)
Type of stroke	Intracerebral hemorrhage	13 (72 %)
	Cerebral infarction	5 (28 %)
Site of lesion	Cerebrum	16 (89 %)
	Brain stem	2 (11 %)
Paralyzed side of lower limb	Right lower limb hemiparesis	12 (67 %)
	Left lower limb hemiparesis	6 (33 %)
Lower limb BRS	Stage III	5 (28 %)
	Stage IV	6 (33 %)
	Stage V	7 (39 %)

[a]$n = 18$

before receiving sham stimulation. The remaining patients received sham stimulation first and had the same interval before receiving high-frequency rTMS (Fig. 5.5). The patients' gait function was assessed before and after each type of stimulation.

The application of high-frequency rTMS involved the use of MagPro R30 and a double cone coil (manufactured by MagVenture) (Fig. 5.6). Ten-second stimulation at 10 Hz was performed every 60 seconds (in other words, at 50-second intervals). This was repeated 20 times within 20 minutes (Fig. 5.7). Stimulation was given to an area on the cranial median line in which the MEP of the tibialis anterior of the unaffected lower limb is most remarkably induced. The intensity of stimulation was set at 90 % of the motor threshold of the tibialis anterior. For sham stimulation, a double cone coil was vertically applied to the same area as in the high-frequency

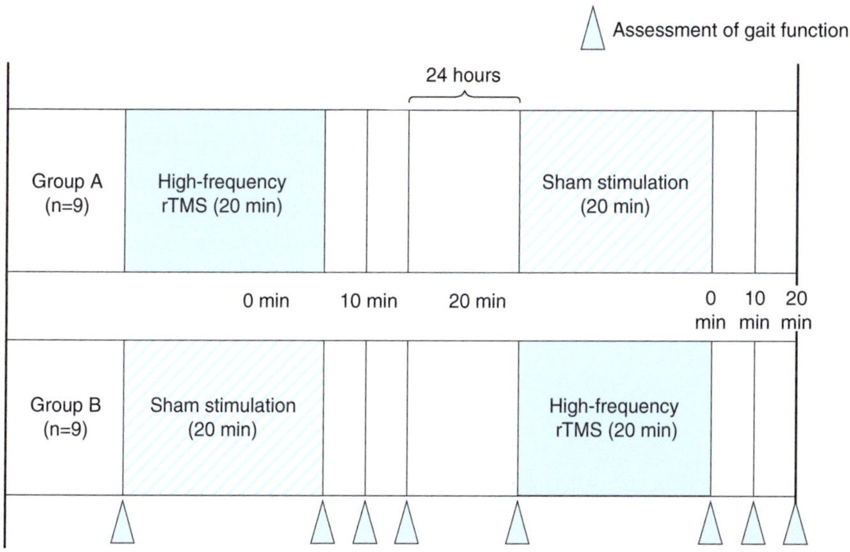

Fig. 5.5 Design of a crossover study. All patients receive both the high-frequency rTMS and sham stimulation for 20 minute each

Fig. 5.6 Application of high-frequency rTMS. A double cone coil is fixed on the cranial median line

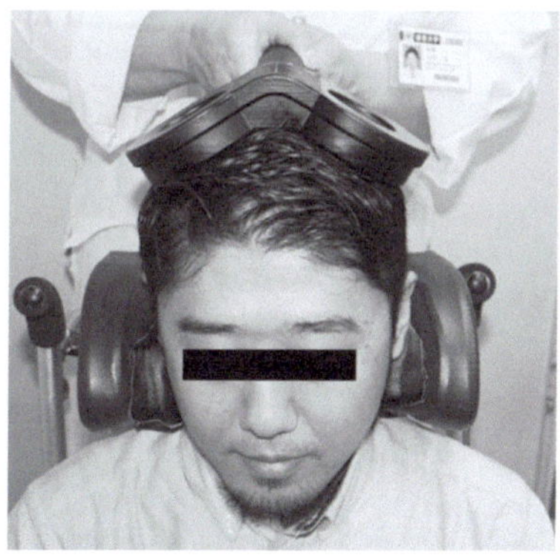

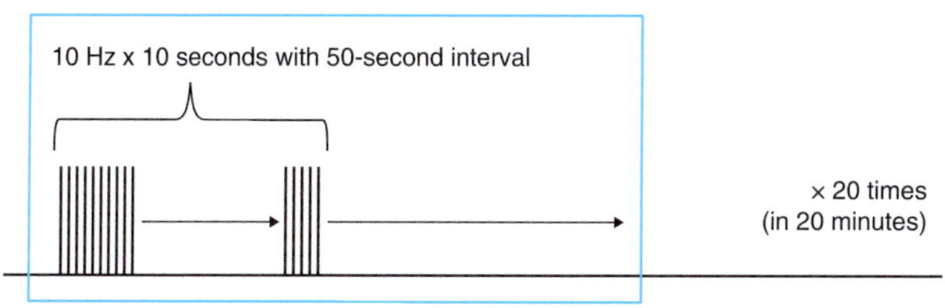

Fig. 5.7 Protocol of high-frequency rTMS. Repeat 10-second stimulation at 10 Hz with 50-second intervals

rTMS so that the coil surface would face forward, not downward. In this way the same stimulation as that in high-frequency rTMS was given for 20 minutes.

Gait function was assessed by determining the walking speed and physiological cost index (PCI) four times: immediately before stimulation, immediately after stimulation, 10 minutes and 20 minutes after completion of stimulation, for each type of stimulation. Walking speed was determined by having a patient walk 10 meters as fast as possible. PCI is an index of gait efficiency, and the smaller the PCI is, the better his/her gait efficiency is considered to be. The study used the following formula [heart rate (beat/minute), walking speed (meter/minute)] to calculate PCI based on the values before and after a 10-meter walk.

C. Results

High-frequency rTMS for 20 minutes was applied to all patients without the incidence of adverse events.

Walking speed was significantly higher in the high-frequency rTMS group than in the sham stimulation group immediately after 20-minute stimulation. The difference remained until 20 minutes after completion of stimulation (Fig. 5.8) [10].

PCI was significantly higher in the high-frequency rTMS group than in the sham stimulation group immediately after stimulation. However, the difference between the groups was not significant at 10 minutes or 20 minutes after completion of stimulation (Fig. 5.9) [10]. As a result of statistical processing, no carryover effect

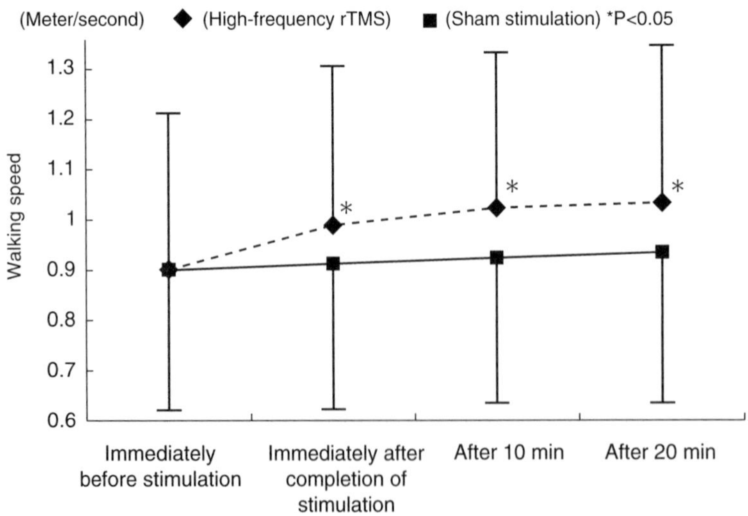

Fig. 5.8 Change in walking speed after stimulation. Walking speed was significantly higher in the high-frequency rTMS group than in the sham stimulation group until 20 minutes after completion of stimulation [10]

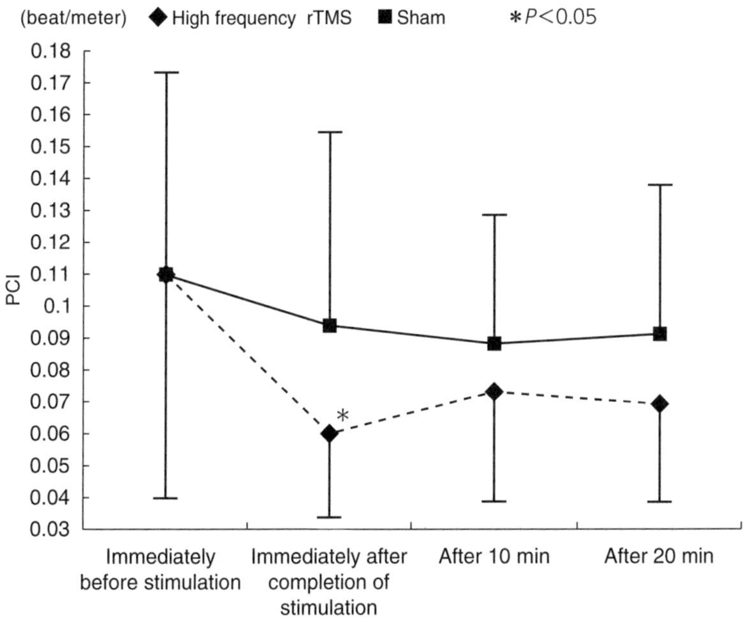

Fig. 5.9 Changes in PCI after stimulation. Only immediately after stimulation was PCI significantly higher in the high-frequency rTMS group than in the sham stimulation group [10]

was recognizable between high-frequency rTMS and sham stimulation. This led to a conclusion that the crossover study had been properly conducted.

These results may be interpreted as a possibility that high-frequency rTMS on the lower limb region of the bilateral primary motor area with the use of a double cone coil may quickly ameliorate the gait function of poststroke patients with hemiparesis. However, the absence of carryover effect between the types of stimulation led to a conclusion that the effects of the 20-minute high-frequency rTMS did not last 24 hours, (predetermined interval between two types of stimulation). One of the reasons why the change in PCI after the application of high-frequency rTMS was transient and its effects were not satisfactory is that PCI, the calculation of which should be based on the heart rate before and after several minutes' walking, was determined before and after only a 10-meter walk. This made changes in the heart rate less likely.

3 Protocol of Combined Use of High-Frequency rTMS and Intensive Physical Therapy

These findings led to the estimation that high-frequency rTMS on the lower limb region of the bilateral primary motor area with the use of a double cone coil would benefit the gait function of stroke patients with lower limb hemiparesis. For

20-minute single rTMS stimulation, however, the possibility that the benefits would not last long was also suggested.

Therefore, we devised a therapeutic protocol for "repeated use of rTMS in combination with intensive physical therapy (PT)," a concept similar to "a combination treatment of rTMS and intensive OT against upper limb hemiparesis (NEURO-15)." In other words, this concept aims at facilitating a functional reorganizing in the lower limb region of the primary motor area by performing high-frequency rTMS with the use of a double cone coil to enhance the plasticity of lower limb region of the bilateral primary motor area before performing intensive PT. The following describes the current facts of efforts for the new combination treatment.

A. Patients

The patients are the same as the abovementioned crossover study. The study enrolled stroke patients with gait disturbance and did not enroll those with severe gait disturbance who always needed a cane or an orthosis and/or had difficulty walking even 10 meters.

B. Methods

The combination treatment was performed as a 13-day protocol for hospitalization treatment (Table 5.3). A concomitant therapy consisting of 20-minute high-frequency rTMS and 60-minute intensive PT was performed in two sessions every day except the day of admission/discharge and Sundays.

Table 5.3 An example of hospitalization schedule for rTMS treatment for lower limb hemiparesis[a]

	Mon.	Tuesday through Saturday	Sun.	Monday through Friday	Sat.
Morning	Admission	High-frequency rTMS (20 minutes)	No treatment	High-frequency rTMS (20 minutes)	Post-treatment evaluation
		Intensive PT (60 minutes)		Intensive PT (60 minutes)	
Afternoon	Pre-treatment evaluation	High-frequency rTMS (20 minutes)		High-frequency rTMS (20 minutes)	Discharge
		Intensive PT (60 minutes)		Intensive PT (60 minutes)	

[a]An example of being hospitalized on Monday

The actual hospitalization schedule is adjusted by each institution

As of December 2012

The application of high-frequency rTMS was the same as in the abovementioned crossover study. In one session, 10-second stimulation at 10 Hz using a double cone coil was repeated 20 times in 20 minutes. The site of stimulation would be the area in which MEP of tibialis anterior of the unaffected lower limb on the cranial median line would most remarkably be induced. The intensity of stimulation would be 90 % of motor threshold of the tibialis (Table 5.4).

One session of intensive PT consisted of one-on-one training session with a physical therapist for 60 minutes. The program included a few minutes of warm-up on the mat, followed by 5–10 minutes of stretching exercise, 5–10 minutes of rising training aimed at increasing muscular strength in the lower limbs, and 25–35 minutes of treadmill training without a relief. Walking speed (exercise intensity) on the treadmill was designed to correspond to Level 4 (somewhat hard) of the modified Borg scale, although this would be adjusted to the patient's gait condition whenever necessary.

C. Results

As of December 2012, the combination treatment has already been performed in more than 20 patients. To date, none of the patients who completed the 13-day protocol experienced any adverse events or adverse reactions of special interest. The protocol was judged to be safe. A comparison between the day of admission and the day of discharge in terms of the effects on gait function suggested improvements in multiple parameters such as walking speed and PCI.

On an individual basis, the amelioration of talipes varus and plantar flexion of the paralyzed lower limb was recognized in many patients. Improvements in toe clearance have also been recognized. Some patients reported subjective changes such as "ease in moving the paralyzed lower limb" and "a feeling that the paralyzed lower limb is lighter than before" (although these were subjective estimations). Substantial differences in walking speed and in the degree of PCI improvement were recognizable among patients.

Table 5.4 An example of hospitalization schedule for rTMS treatment for lower limb hemiparesis[a]

Coil used	Double cone coil
Site	Bilateral cerebrum (lower limb region of the primary motor area)
Intensity	90 % of motor threshold
Frequency	High-frequency rTMS (10 Hz)
Duration	1 session lasting 20 minutes (2000 pulses), twice daily
No. of days at hosp.	13 days

[a]The actual treatment is adjusted by each institution

As of December 2012

4 Future Challenges

As mentioned, high-frequency rTMS on the lower limb region of the bilateral primary motor area using a double cone coil may be a beneficial means of therapeutic intervention in poststroke lower limb hemiparesis. At this point, however, establishing this as a therapeutic intervention requires at least the following issues to be solved.

1) Intensity of rTMS

The study determined the intensity of rTMS based on the motor threshold of the tibialis anterior of the nonparalyzed lower limb. This procedure would make it possible to determine the motor threshold and the intensity of stimulation in almost all patients. In a condition such as serious damage to the nerve pathway connecting the lesional hemisphere to the paralyzed lower limb, the stimulation may be insufficient (too weak) against the primary motor area of the lesional hemisphere. Because of this, the determination of intensity of stimulation may also require consideration of the motor threshold of the muscle of the paralyzed lower limb.

2) Details of the PT Program for Combined Use with rTMS

At present, we use the PT program, the core of which is gait training on a treadmill, in combination with high-frequency rTMS. It is quite possible that this training program is not optimal. For example, increasing the proportion of an exercise for strengthening the lower limb muscles would be better. Determining "a more optimal PT program" for combined use with rTMS would help increase the benefits of rTMS.

3) Introduction of a Gait Analysis

The recent study showed that the application of high-frequency rTMS using a double cone coil would ameliorate gait function. However, the mechanism has yet to be elucidated. Doing so may require a gait analysis and a motion analysis to be performed over time.

4) Application of Brain Function Imaging

It may be expected that the amelioration of the gait function after the application of high-frequency rTMS using a double cone coil will be followed by a certain plastic change in the lower limb region of the primary motor area or its surrounding tissue.

However, this has not been searched by brain function imaging such as functional MRI (fMRI) and PET.

5) Necessity of a Randomized Controlled Trial

Showing evidence of the usefulness of concomitant therapy with high-frequency rTMS and intensive PT requires RCT to compare the "high-frequency rTMS + intensive PT group" and "sham stimulation + intensive PT group."

The rTMS treatment for gait disturbances induced by poststroke lower limb hemiparesis is still in a developmental stage and needs further improvement. As far as our findings suggest, however, it is quite possible that the application of high-frequency rTMS using a double cone coil to the lower limb region of the primary motor area becomes one of the new treatment options for lower limb hemiparesis and gait disturbances.

Appendix: Intensive Physical Therapy That Should Be Used in Combination with rTMS

Lower Limb Dysfunction and PT in Poststroke Hemiparesis

The following discusses a mechanism that may occur if rTMS on an upper limb has influenced lower limb function.

In PT, the severity of poststroke hemiparesis is determined by the Brunnstrom recovery stages (BRS) (Table 5.5) [12, 13]. The staging is intended to facilitate judgment on whether or not a limb can move and perform isolated movement. In a normal condition of "isolation," the person can do a simple exercise and move his/her hands, legs, and fingers independently at will. Separation can be an important criterion to decide whether a limb is in a normal condition. Nonisolation does not always mean a state in which a limb cannot move at all.

In BRS, Stage IV or higher means isolation is recognizable. However, it is hard to discern the conceptual reduction of spasticity from the expression of isolation. Judgments as rule of thumb cannot be ruled out. If the muscle tone has increased, it is often the case that the expression of isolation is inadequate. In particular, it has much to do with factors such as posture, action, and move. Under load, abnormality of muscle tone uniformly becomes apparent. Differences between Stage IV and V should be decided by observing the same joint movement performed in different postures. In other words, this means isolation is strongly influenced by an increase in postural muscle tone.

The postural muscle tone allows a hemiparesis patient to move the upper limb, which is relatively relaxed in a supine position, to take a specific posture in the upright position or while walking.

This is the so-called Wernicke-Mann leg position. Its characteristics are more apparent in a sitting position than in a supine position and while walking than while

Table 5.5 Brunnstrom recovery stage (lower limbs and trunk)

Stage	Lower limbs and trunk
I	[Flaccidity] Neither muscle contraction nor movement is possible reflexively or voluntarily
II	[Spasticity occurrence period] Muscle contraction occurs from an associative reaction or voluntarily (elements of synergy slightly occur)
III	[Remarkable spasticity] Synergy or some of its elements occurs voluntarily. Synergy with flexion and extension
IV	[Spasticity slightly reduced] A patient can do an exercise that is slightly separated from synergy In a sitting position, a patient can flex the knee by 90 degrees or more and slide the sole backward along the floor In a sitting position, a patient can dorsiflex the foot with the heel remaining in contact with the floor
V	[Spasticity reduced] A patient can do an exercise that is considerably separated from synergy In an standing position, a patient can place the hip joint in an extended position and flex the knees In an standing position, a patient can extend the foot slightly forward and dorsiflex the ankle joint with the heel remaining in contact with the floor
VI	[Minimum spasticity] In an standing position, a patient can abduct the hip joint while keeping the knee extended In a sitting position, a patient can alternately contract the inner and outer knee flexors

Excerpted from Refs. [12] and [13]

sitting. An increase in the muscle tone in the upper limb influences movements of the trunk and lower limbs.

A gait of a human being is phylogenetically differentiated from that of other vertebrates by the movement of the trunk when crawling on hands and knees. This can be explained, in an arthrokinematic manner, as a smooth and alternate rolling and sliding movement based on the retention of centripetal force, and kinematically as a phase movement where the limbs swing alternately. When an upper limb swings forward, the lower limb on the opposite side makes a step forward. When an upper limb swings backward, the lower limb on the opposite side is guided to the toe-off position through the stance phase. In other words, a gait consists of regular movements in which upper limbs and lower limbs move in opposite phases. A forward movement is accompanied by an axial rotation around the trunk (Fig. 5.10).

Opposite phases with left-right alternate movements require the upper limbs to swing and the lower limbs to take a step. The more poststroke hemiparesis makes isolation insufficient, the more it strategically supplements a compensatory function that replaces the functions of the upper limbs and trunk that are necessary for walking. Worse, abnormality in muscle tone makes it hard to form a smooth cycle. As a consequence the gait cannot be symmetrical, and the gait of the patient with stroke takes on characteristic patterns such as extension thrust pattern (a pattern in which

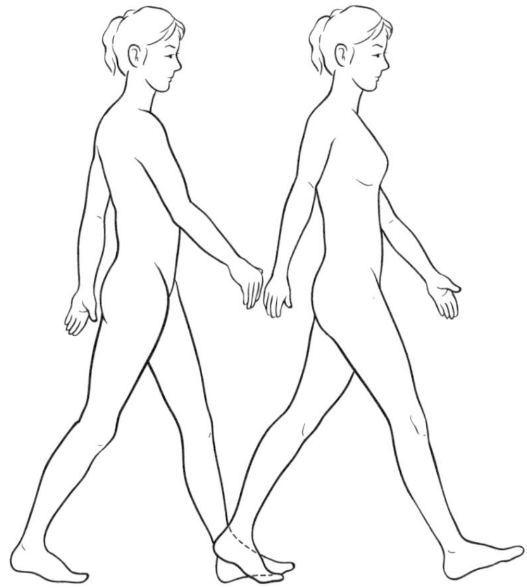

Fig. 5.10 Opposite phases of a human gait. When the left leg makes a step forward, the right hand swings forward. When the right leg makes a step forward, the left hand swings forward

the knee is overextended), stiff knee pattern (a pattern in which a stiff knee results in less flexion), and bucking knee pattern (a pattern in which the knee is overflexed). An abnormal gait pattern lacks efficiency and burdens the cardiopulmonary function. As a consequence, the patient slows walking speed to stabilize, and the possibility of secondary complications such as falls and pain increases.

Here, it is worth noting that the effects of rTMS treatment demonstrated by Abo et al. [14–18] through a study with a rat model can be explained as follows: functional compensation in the lesional hemisphere and in the residual regions around the lesion, not in the nonlesional hemisphere on the nonlesional side, plays an important role in the partial involvement within an adult's brain that concerns recovery from paralysis. For tissues around the lesion of the affected brain that are considered to facilitate functional recovery, low-frequency stimulation on the nonlesional hemisphere is reported to have reduced interhemispheric inhibition and activated functional compensation.

In fact, the effects of rTMS on upper limb hemiparesis are reported. Given the above mechanism of a human gait, the effects of rTMS on reducing muscle tone in the upper limbs may also bring about a change in gait that requires coordination of the upper and lower limbs.

Usefulness of Treadmill Gait Training

A gait is an unconscious movement and is based on a reflexive mechanism. It is considered that a gait can be divided into three different phases as a stratified control (Fig. 5.11) [19]. The first phase involves planning and preparation for movements in the cerebrocortical motor area. The second phase involves coordination by the brain stem. The third phase is characterized by control by the central pattern generator (CPG) consisting of a group of spinal interneurons. CPG does not involve voluntary control by the cerebrum and is coordinated in a reflexive manner. While walking, a person does not think about when to move the other leg forward every time he or she takes a step. Every step is not based on intentional adaptation to a command to contact the ground or floor with a heel. Voluntary control by the cerebrum is limited to adaptation to a signal or changes in road surface, unevenness of the floor or ground, and similar.

When walking on a flat surface, a patient with hemiparesis moves a leg forward and contacts the ground or floor with a good clearance and keeps the feet supporting the body to prevent falls, before shifting his/her center of gravity toward the opposite side, the nonparalyzed lower limb. While walking, a patient with hemiparesis remains conscious about these procedures. In particular, consciousness about these procedures is greater in patients with problems such as sensory impairment, weakened muscle strength in the nonparalyzed lower limb, and fear that comes from advanced age. These people are more likely to stop walking before stepping over a bump or passing someone. Many of these people walk asymmetrically by leaning the trunk forward and leaning the pelvis backward to flex the hip joint with a center of gravity on the nonparalyzed lower limb. Even the coordination of pace is based on the patient's will. It is not always the case that doing a lot of walking every day will facilitate recovery. To induce a qualitative

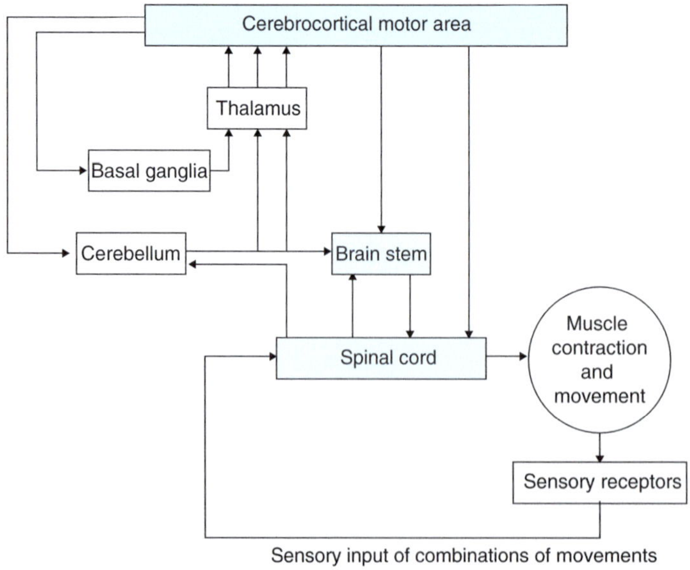

Fig. 5.11 Diagram of stratified control [8]

effect, a physical therapist gives visual stimulation with the use of oral instructions, a mirror or a video, shows changes in time-distance factors, and combines them with handling in an effort to bring about alteration. In fact, the authors do this in clinical practice. It is difficult to scientifically verify this type of intervention in a gait.

On the other hand, walking on a treadmill involves the floor surface shifting backward at a constant speed, providing a kind of gait using passive stepping. In terms of floor reaction force waveform overall, walking on a treadmill involves greater similarity than walking on a flat surface does [20]. Despite differences in minor parameters, it is considered to be possible to diagnose and determine the degree of amelioration of gait disturbances with the use of a treadmill [21].

For a period of time after starting a treadmill, the patient continues to focus on movements (stimulation) on the floor surface and may feel insecure at times. Since the treadmill gait training is provided in a stepwise manner, the patient gradually adapts him/herself to the changeless and constant stimulation. This may facilitate a shift from the conscious movements of legs to unconscious movements. This is a clear difference from walking on a flat surface where stimulation occurs randomly and in many different forms. It is also important that the treadmill gait training ensures physical therapists sufficient time for observation.

Studies of paraparesis induced by spinal cord injury have confirmed some effects of walking on a treadmill. For example, walking on a treadmill may exert effects in the form of induction of muscle activity in harmony with a walking cycle [22] or achievement of a hip extension position in the late stance phase [23]. In addition, using a treadmill serves as an opportunity for a hemiparesis patient to become aware of a left-right gap in his/her gait cycle. In patients whose muscle tone in the upper limb has been reduced after rTMS, using a treadmill may influence upper limb swings and the rotation of a trunk and, consequently, make it possible to swing a lower limb and to achieve a standing position within an area of hip joint extension. Compared with walking on a flat surface that is a patient-steering movement, walking on a treadmill is a passive movement adapted to an automatically moving surface. The use of a treadmill may be expected to help improve ambulatory ability through the indirect effects of reduction of muscle tone in the upper limbs and trunk, provided that rTMS has reduced the tension in the upper limbs and made it easier for isolation to express.

In today's healthcare and welfare practices, aggressive PT is becoming increasingly hard to perform with patients in the maintenance period. Many patients engage in self-exercise as a part of their daily life. The Japanese Guidelines for the Management of Stroke 2009 [24] recommends rising and walking for rehabilitation in the maintenance period. However, it is hard for a patient alone to concentrate on a specific instruction without receiving advice. This is especially true for patients with hemiparesis in the generation to which long-term care insurance services do not apply. We hope that rTMS will play the role of a means of preconditioning in performing intensive PT for patients who continue training on their own.

References

1. Jørgensen HS, Nakayama H, Raaschou HO, et al. Recovery of walking function in stroke patients; the Copenhagen Stroke Study. Arch Phys Med Rehabil. 1995;76:27–32.
2. Abo M, Kakuda W. Rehabilitation for cerebrovascular disease. Nihon Ishikai Zasshi. 2011;140:31–5. Japanese.
3. Chen R, Cohen LG, Hallett M. Role of the ipsilateral motor cortex in voluntary movement. Can J Neurol Sci. 1997;24:284–91.
4. Luft AR, Smith GV, Forrester L, et al. Comparing brain activation associated with isolated upper and lower limb movement across corresponding joints. Hum Brain Mapp. 2002;17:131–40.
5. Luft AR, Forrester L, Macko RF, et al. Brain activation of lower extremity movement in chronically impaired stroke survivors. Neuroimage. 2005;26:184–94.
6. Enzinger C, Dawes H, Johansen-Berg H, et al. Brain activity changes associated with treadmill training after stroke. Stroke. 2009;40:2460–7.
7. Yen CL, Wang RY, Liao KK, et al. Gait training induced change in corticomotor excitability in patients with chronic stroke. Neurorehabil Neural Repair. 2008;22:22–30.
8. Stokić DS, McKay WB, Scott L, et al. Intracortical inhibition of lower limb motor-evoked potentials after paired transcranial magnetic stimulation. Exp Brain Res. 1997;117:437–43.
9. Terao Y, Ugawa Y, Hanajima R, et al. Predominant activation of I1-waves from the leg motor area by transcranial magnetic stimulation. Brain Res. 2000;859:137–46.
10. Kakuda W, Abo M, Nakayama Y, et al. High-frequency rTMS using a double cone coil for gait disturbance. Acta Neurol Scand 7 Feb 2013.
11. Wassermann EM. Risk and safety of repetitive transcranial magnetic stimulation; report and suggested guidelines from the international workshop on the safety of repetitive transcranial magnetic stimulation, June 5–7, 1996. Electroencephalogr Clin Neurophysiol. 1998;108:1–16.
12. Brunnstrom S. Movement therapy in hemiplegia. New York: Harper and Row; 1970.
13. Fukui K, Fujita T, Miyasaka M, et al. Stroke frontier: from acute phase diagnosis to rehabilitation. 4th ed. Tokyo: Ishiyaku Pub; 2009. p. 85. Japanese.
14. Abo M, Chen Z, Lai LJ, et al. Functional recovery after brain lesion; contralateral neuromodulation; an fMRI study. Neuroreport. 2001;12:1543–7.
15. Abo M, Yamauchi H, Chen Z, et al. Behavioural recovery correlated with MRI in a rat experimental stroke model. Brain Inj. 2003;17:799–808.
16. Abo M, Suzuki M, Senoo A, et al. Influence of isoflurane concentration and hypoxia on functional magnetic resonance imaging for the detection of bicuculline-induced neuronal activation. Neurosignals. 2004;13:144–9.
17. Takata K, Yamauchi H, Tatsuno H, et al. Is the ipsilateral cortex surrounding the lesion or the non-injured contralateral cortex important for motor recovery in rats with photochemically induced cortical lesions? Eur Neurol. 2006;56:106–12.
18. Abo M, Yamauchi H, Suzuki M, et al. Facilitated beam-walking recovery during acute phase by kynurenic acid treatment in a rat model of photochemically induced thrombosis causing focal cerebral ischemia. Neurosignals. 2006–2007;15:102–10.
19. Nakazawa K. Neurorehabilitation of walking: theoretical and clinical goals to regain walking. Tokyo: Kyorin-Shoin; 2010. p. 57. Japanese.
20. Okada M, Sakurai H, Suzuki Y, et al. Comparison of ground reaction forces between overground and treadmill walking. J Jpn Phys Ther Assoc. 2002;29:209–17. Japanese.
21. Sakurai H, Sonoda S, Okada M, et al. Gait analysis using a treadmill: comparison of kinetic parameters among various walking velocity settings. Jpn J Clin Neurophysiol. 2002;30:315–9. Japanese.
22. Dietz V, Colombo G, Jensen L. Locomotor activity in spinal man. Lancet. 1994;344:1260–3.
23. Nakazawa K, Kawashima N, Kawashima N, et al. Induction of locomotor-like EMG activity in paraplegic persons by orthotic gait training. Exp Brain Res. 2004;157:117–23.
24. Shinohara Y, Ogawa S, et al. Japanese guidelines for the management of stroke. Kyowa Kikaku. 2009;2009:308–12.

Chapter 6
rTMS in the Acute Phase of Stroke

Introduction

There are many reports on the effectiveness of repetitive transcranial magnetic stimulation (rTMS) for the treatment of stroke worldwide, and in recent years rTMS has become the most promising field of neurohabilitation. However, the overwhelming majority of these reports are on the application of rTMS for the treatment of upper extremity paralysis in the chronic phase of stroke, and there are only few reports on studies in which rTMS was used in acute stroke patients (Table 6.1) [1–13]. There are two main reasons why research on the use of rTMS for the treatment of acute stroke patients still lags. One is safety, namely, the fear of epileptic seizures, which is one of the risks that are associated with rTMS therapy. Epileptic seizures in acute stroke are an independent prognostic factor for in-hospital mortality, and therefore a cautious evaluation of the appropriateness of rTMS application is required [14]. Another reason is the study design. Obviously, spontaneous recovery plays an important role in acute stroke, and therefore for detecting the effects of rTMS it is necessary that patients are selected based on strict criteria or that the study is conducted with a large number of patients. Moreover, such studies must have a randomized controlled trial (RCT) or a crossover trial (COT) study design. In recent years, there has been a tendency to question whether therapeutic intervention studies that are expected to be highly beneficial are ethically justifiable as far as the control group is concerned, when they are conducted as a RCT. Meanwhile, COTs extend the intervention period and therefore can be said not to be suited as a clinical research method in acute hospitals that aim to shorten the duration of hospitalization.

The difficulty of conducting therapeutic intervention studies that involve acute stroke patients is not limited to rTMS alone. In a review by Stinear et al. from 2013, only 30 intervention studies on the rehabilitation (in the following referred as reha) of motor disorders after acute stroke are rated as high-quality studies, and it is described that there are only 5 research papers on rTMS, including a research paper

M. Abo, W. Kakuda, *Rehabilitation with rTMS*,
DOI 10.1007/978-3-319-20982-1_6

Table 6.1 List of rTMS intervention studies for acute phase of stroke to date [1–13]

Authors	Year of publication	Number of subjects	Summary
Khedr EM, et al. [1]	2005	26	ADL was improved by rTMS
Liepert J, et al. [2]	2007	20	Upper limb function was improved by rTMS of 1 Hz
Di Lazzaro V, et al. [3]	2008	12	The activity of the cerebral cortex on the lesional side was enhanced by either cTBS or iTBS
Khedr EM, et al. [4]	2009	36	Upper limb function was improved by rTMS of 1 and 3 Hz. In particular, the improvement lasted until three months later when rTMS of 1 Hz was performed
Khedr EM, et al. [5]	2010	48	Upper limb function was improved by rTMS of 1 and 3 Hz
Khedr EM, et al. [6]	2010	22	Dysphagia due to the brainstem infarction was improved by rTMS of 3 Hz and the improvement lasted until two months later
Khaleel SH, et al. [7]	2010	31	The cerebral blood flow in the MCA region was improved by rTMS of 10 Hz over DLPFC
Chang WH, et al. [8]	2010	28	Upper and lower limb motor function and ADL were improved by rTMS of 10 Hz
Hsu YF, et al. [9]	2013	12	Upper limb function was improved by iTBS
Sasaki N, et al. [10]	2013	29	Upper limb function was improved by rTMS of 1 and 10 Hz. In particular, greater improvement was observed when rTMS of 10 Hz was performed
Kim BR, et al. [11]	2013	27	As a result of comparing the effect of rTMS of 1 and 10 Hz over USN, improvement was observed when rTMS of 10 Hz was performed
Kim WS, et al. [12]	2014	32	Balance was improved in patients with cerebellar ataxia when rTMS of 1 Hz was performed
Sasaki N, et al. [13]	2014	58	Upper limb function improved further when rTMS of 1 and 10 Hz was performed simultaneously than when only rTMS of 10 Hz was performed

rTMS repetitive transcranial magnetic stimulation, *cTBS* continuous theta-burst stimulation, *iTBS* intermittent theta-burst stimulation, *DLPFC* dorsolateral prefrontal cortex, *MCA* middle cerebral artery, *ADL* ability of daily living, *USN* unilateral spatial neglect

by the authors [15]. However, all consider the effectiveness of rTMS in acute stroke patients to be positive, and also the meta-analysis by Hsu et al. showed that the effectiveness of rTMS when used for improving upper extremity paralysis is higher in acute stroke than in chronic stroke patients (effect size: chronic stroke 0.66, acute stroke 0.79) [16]. In this report we will briefly introduce the results of two studies on the use of rTMS for the treatment of upper extremity paralysis in acute stroke patients that we reported to date.

Which rTMS Modality Is More Beneficial for Acute Stroke, High- or Low-Frequency rTMS?

I will reserve details on the principles of rTMS for a future occasion. In short, there are basically two types of rTMS, stimulatory high-frequency rTMS (HF-rTMS) and inhibitory low-frequency rTMS (LF-rTMS). For the treatment of upper extremity paralysis in the chronic phase of stroke the following rTMS methods can be used. A method that improves paralysis by enhancing the activity of the lesional hemisphere through interhemispheric inhibition (IHI) resulting from inhibition of the overactivity of the nonlesional hemisphere, which can be achieved by applying LF-rTMS (this method is similar to the NovEl Intervention Using Repetitive TMS and Intensive Occupational Therapy [NEURO] [17] that is conducted at the Department of Rehabilitation Medicine of Jikei University School of Medicine), and a method that directly activates the lesional hemisphere by applying HF-rTMS (Fig. 6.1). First we examined the effectiveness of these two types of rTMS when used for the treatment of upper extremity paralysis in acute stroke patients [10].

1) Patients and Methods

This study involved 29 patients with newly developed acute-stage cerebral infarction or cerebral hemorrhage (mean age at the time of hospitalization: 65 ± 10 years old, 13 cerebral infarction, 16 cerebral hemorrhage) who had lesions in the unilateral

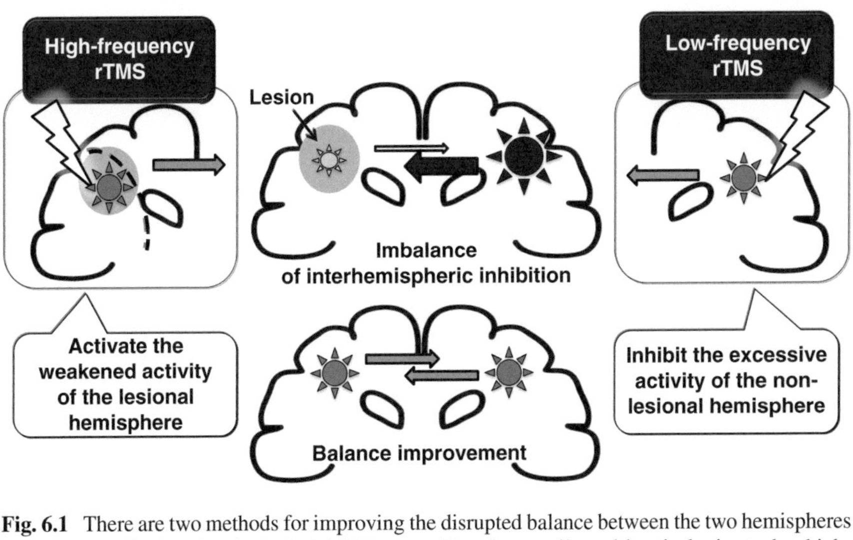

Fig. 6.1 There are two methods for improving the disrupted balance between the two hemispheres that is caused by interhemispheric inhibition resulting from unilateral hemispheric stroke: high-frequency rTMS (HF-rTMS) for activating the decreased function of the lesional hemisphere and low-frequency rTMS (LF-rTMS) for inhibiting the overactivity of the nonlesional hemisphere

middle cerebral artery territory that did not include the cortex. Patients hospitalized 6 hours or more after the onset of stroke, patients who had been administered tissue plasminogen activator (tPA), patients who had undergone surgery, and patients with severe disturbance of consciousness were excluded from the study. Subjects were randomly allocated to the HF-rTMS group (9 subjects), LF-rTMS group (11 subjects), and sham stimulation group (9 subjects), and within 30 days after onset of stroke (mean 17.4±5.4 days), 1 stimulation session was conducted each day for 5 consecutive days as described below. During these 5 days before and after intervention changes in the grasping power (GP) of the paralyzed hand and fingers, and tapping frequency (TAP) within 30 seconds were compared between the 3 groups.

2) Application of rTMS

The site at which maximum flexion of the contralateral index finger was achieved following primary motor cortex stimulation through single-pulse TMS was set as rTMS stimulation site, and stimulation intensity was set at 90 % of the minimum stimulation intensity at which index finger flexion was achieved. During 1 session, in the HF-rTMS group 10-Hz rTMS trains were applied for 10 seconds to the stimulation site on the lesional side followed by a pause of 50 seconds, and this was repeated 10 times. In the LF-rTMS group 1-Hz rTMS trains were applied for 30 minutes to the stimulation site on the nonlesional side. In the sham stimulation group a stimulation coil was placed vertically toward the skull surface in such a way that no magnetic flux penetrated the brain, and the nonlesional hemisphere was stimulated at a frequency of 1 Hz (so that only the sound of stimulation could be heard) for 10 minutes.

3) Results

Prior to intervention there were no differences between the three groups regarding the clinical characteristics of the patients, stroke severity, or severity of paralysis. No adverse events were observed in any of the patients who participated in this study, and the study protocol could be completed. During the 5 days of intervention no significant changes in GP and TAP were observed in the sham stimulation group; however, in both the HF-rTMS group and the LF-rTMS group a significant improvement of GP and TAP was observed (Fig. 6.2). GP was 0.6±0.7 kg in the sham stimulation group, 4.2±2.8 kg in the HF-rTMS group, and 2.3±2.9 kg in the LF-rTMS group, and thus when comparing the increase in GP among these three groups, in the HF-rTMS group a significantly greater increase in GP was observed than in the sham stimulation group. TAP was 2.8±4.1 times in the sham stimulation group, 12.3±8.7 times in the HF-rTMS group, and 14.3±15.1 times in the LF-rTMS group, and thus also the increase in TAP was significantly greater in the HF-rTMS group than in the sham stimulation group (Fig. 6.3).

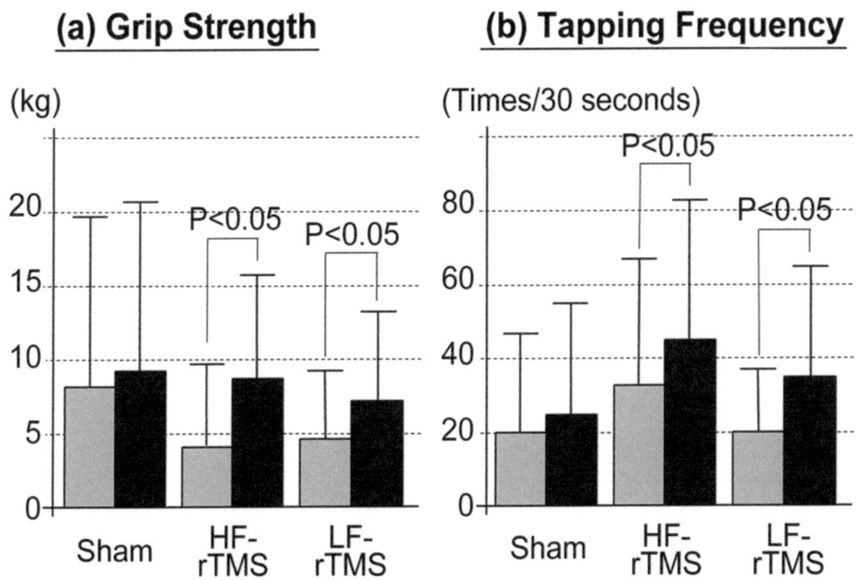

Fig. 6.2 When comparing grip strength and tapping frequency before and after rTMS intervention for a period of 5 days, in the sham stimulation group no significant improvement was observed either for grip strength or for tapping frequency; however, in both the HF-rTMS group and LF-rTMS group a significant improvement was observed for both grip strength and tapping frequency

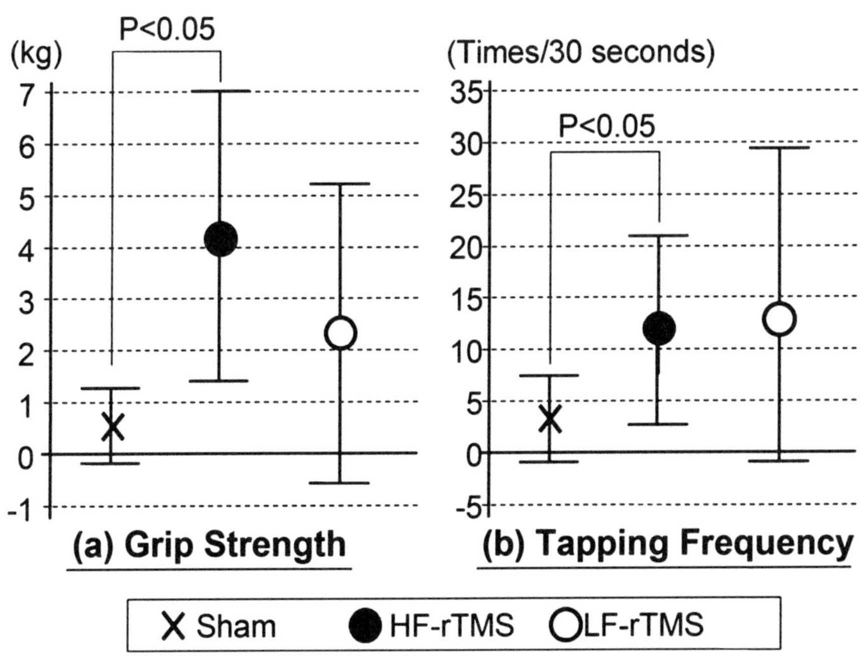

Fig. 6.3 A comparison of changes in grip strength and tapping frequency following rTMS intervention for a period of 5 days showed that only in the HF-rTMS group changes in grip strength and tapping frequency were significantly greater than in the sham group

Is Bilateral rTMS More Beneficial for Acute Stroke than High-Frequency rTMS?

Next, we thought that probably a stronger effect could be achieved if HF-rTMS and LF-rTMS were applied simultaneously and devised a method for conducting bilateral rTMS (BL-rTMS) by using two rTMS devices. Then we compared the results obtained with BL-rTMS and those obtained with unilateral HF-rTMS, which showed better results than the other stimulation methods in the previous study described above [13].

1) Patients and Methods

This study involved 58 patients with acute-stage cerebral infarction or cerebral hemorrhage who fulfilled the same criteria as those in the previous study described above (mean age at the time of hospitalization: 65 ± 10 years old, 36 cerebral infarction, 22 cerebral hemorrhage). Subjects were randomly allocated to 2 groups, the BL-rTMS group (27 subjects) and the LF-rTMS group (31 subjects). The period until the start of intervention was set at within 15 days after onset of symptoms (mean 9.7 ± 3.3 days), and thus was shorter than in the previous study. In all subjects one stimulation session was conducted each day for 5 consecutive days as described below. During these 5 days before and after intervention changes in the Brunnstrom Recovery Stage (BRS) of the upper limb and hand-finger, GP, and TAP were compared between the two groups.

2) Application of rTMS

Stimulation site and intensity were set in the same way as in Study 1. In the HF-rTMS group 10-Hz rTMS trains were applied for 10 seconds to the stimulation site on the lesional side followed by a pause of 50 seconds, and this was repeated 10 times. In the BL-rTMS group rTMS was conducted by applying 1-Hz rTMS trains for 10 minutes to the stimulation site on the nonlesional side, followed by 10-Hz rTMS trains that were applied for 10 seconds to the stimulation site on the lesional side, and 1-Hz rTMS trains that were applied for 50 seconds to the stimulation site on the nonlesional side, and this was repeated 10 times alternately.

3) Results

Prior to intervention there were no differences between the two groups regarding the clinical characteristics of the patients, stroke severity, or severity of paralysis. No adverse events were observed in any of the patients who participated in this study, and the study protocol could be completed. During the 5 days of intervention, both in the BL-rTMS group and the HF-rTMS group a significant improvement in the BRS of the upper limb and hand-finger, GP, and TAP was observed (Table 6.2). Although increases in GP and TAP tended to be higher in the BL-rTMS group, no significant differences were observed. However, the amount of improvement of paralysis was more pronounced in the BL-rTMS group, namely, the amount of improvement in BRS of the upper limb was 1.4 ± 0.9 in the BL-rTMS group compared to 0.7 ± 0.7 in the HF-rTMS group, and the amount of improvement in BRS of the hand-finger was 1.4 ± 0.8 in the BL-rTMS group compared to 0.7 ± 0.7 in the HF-rTMS group, and thus in either case a more significant improvement was observed in the BL-rTMS group than in the HF-rTMS group (Fig. 6.4).

Interpretation of Our Study Results

This series of studies demonstrated that rTMS is also effective for the treatment of upper extremity paralysis in the acute phase of stroke, that in particular HF-rTMS is highly effective, and that through BL-rTMS, namely, the simultaneous conduct of HF-rTMS and LF-rTMS, even better results can be expected.

As noted, different from the chronic phase of stroke, spontaneous recovery is an important factor in acute stroke, and for this very reason it is necessary to set up a control group in the study design. We know from experience that a very large number of patients "have the feeling" that their condition improved even if only a coil was placed on their head. It is also conceivable that it actually affects the treatment outcome, and therefore it is desirable to conduct sham stimulation in the control group. Taking this into consideration, we conducted RCT in the first study (Study 1) in all three groups, namely, in the LF-rTMS, HF-rTMS, and sham stimulation group. In Study 2 no sham group was set up, and therefore this was only a pilot study that arose based on the results of Study 1. However, the criteria for participating in this study and the conditions for conducting HF-rTMS were the same as in Study 1.

The rationale for applying LF-rTMS in the treatment of upper extremity paralysis in the chronic phase of stroke is the overactivity of the nonlesional hemisphere, and the enhanced inhibition of the lesional hemisphere that is caused by unbalances that result from IHI [18]. This is the greatest problem that rTMS procedures must be determined distinctively for acute and chronic stroke. In short, the crucial question is when this imbalance in brain activity will occur. In the study by Marshall et al., in which functional MRI (fMRI) was used, it was shown that although brain activity of the nonlesional side was not notably enhanced in the acute phase after stroke, it was significantly enhanced after several months [19]. If that is the case, then one might not be able to expect that in acute stroke a decrease in the activity of the nonlesional hemisphere that is achieved by LF-rTMS will result in the appropriate release of the inhibited lesional hemisphere. One could also say that the results of the first study

Table 6.2 Changes in upper limb function before and after performing rTMS in Study 2

	BL-rTMS				HF-rTMS			
	Pre-intervention	Post-intervention	Change in the value	statistics	Pre-intervention	Post-intervention	Change in the value	Statistics
BRS of upper limb	2.9 (1.4)	4.3 (1.5)	1.4 (0.9)	<0.01	2.8 (1.4)	3.5 (1.5)	0.7 (0.7)	<0.01
BRS of hand-fingers	3.0 (1.6)	4.4 (1.6)	1.4 (0.8)	<0.01	2.6 (1.5)	3.3 (1.6)	0.7 (0.7)	<0.01
Grip strength, kg	4.8 (7.6)	8.4 (9.5)	3.6 (3.6)	<0.01	3.1 (5.7)	5.7 (8.2)	2.6 (3.7)	<0.01
Tapping frequency, times/30 seconds	23.6 (24.6)	36.5 (27.0)	12.9 (9.9)	<0.01	18.4 (25.0)	28.3 (30.1)	9.9 (10.7)	<0.01

BRS Brunnstrom recovery stage

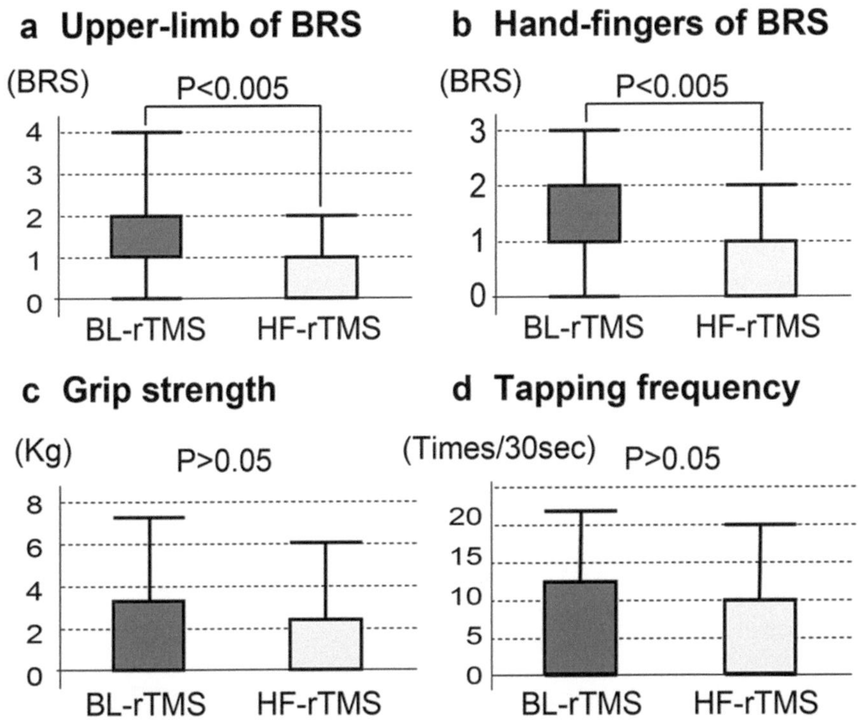

Fig. 6.4 When conducting rTMS intervention for a period of 5 days, significantly larger changes in the BRS of the upper limb and hand-finger were observed in the BL-rTMS group than in the HF-rTMS group. However, no differences in grip strength and tapping frequency were observed between the two groups

indirectly support that there is not much overactivity of the nonlesional hemisphere during the acute stage.

We think that as long as patients cannot be treated in an environment where functional brain imaging tests such as fMRI can be conducted for assessing individual brain activity, at present the most appropriate treatment method is BL-rTMS, which was conducted in the second study. Presumably, brain activity changes over time in various ways depending among other things on the size and site of the lesion, and the age of the patient. However, when applying BL-rTMS it is possible to take a direct approach with which both hemispheres can be treated simultaneously, regardless of the state of balance in the activity levels of the lesional and nonlesional hemisphere. The simultaneous application of two types of stimulation is expected to have a synergetic effect on both sides of the brain that is mediated by the IHI. This method has already been reported also to be used for the treatment of upper extremity paralysis in the chronic phase of stroke, and has been shown to be more effective than unilateral stimulation [20]. If there are any problems regarding BL-rTMS then these are the stimulation intensity and the number of stimuli. Moreover, obviously it is assumed that the unilateral application of HF-rTMS or LF-rTMS will also increase the risk of epileptic seizures. However, similar to previous reports on the application of BL-rTMS in the chronic phase of stroke, when we used the study protocol for the treatment of acute stroke not a single patient dropped out from the study, and no side effects or adverse effects were observed. The optimal number of stimuli and the limit of its application are issues that are related to rTMS in general and require further verification over a longer period of time.

In addition, an important difference between the acute and the chronic phase of stroke is the plasticity of the brain. Gao et al. reported that in an intervention study, in which they conducted rTMS in acute stroke in a rat model of cerebral infarction, they could prevent the progression of lesions more significantly in the group in which HF-rTMS was conducted than in the group in which sham stimulation was conducted [21]. This suggests that HF-rTMS exerts effects that prevent the death of neurons. At this stage it is not clear whether LF-rTMS has the same effect; however, when considering that according to the Hebbian Learning Rule the firing rate of neurons affects the number of synaptic connections, then it is conceivable that direct stimulatory stimulation of the lesional cortex can be expected to be more effective than the reduction of excessive inhibition that is mediated by the IHI. We think that at present, from the viewpoint of brain plasticity as well, in many patients rTMS in acute stroke would be more effective, if it were conducted on the basis of HF-rTMS that is applied to the lesional hemisphere.

Future Challenges of rTMS for Acute Stroke

Although there are reports that rTMS is applied not only for upper extremity paralysis in the chronic phase of stroke but also for various symptoms such as paralysis of the lower extremity, alogia, other higher brain dysfunctions, dysphagia, and ataxia, there are still only very few reports on the application of rTMS in acute stroke, and the fields of application are only limited. Taking together the findings that were made to date, there are many cases in which methods that are effective in the chronic phase of stroke are also effective in acute stroke without having to be changed. We therefore think that after a treatment method was confirmed to be effective and safe in the chronic phase of stroke, it is possible to immediately move on to studies that apply this method in acute stroke. In fact, a future challenge is to search for a strategy that is effective in acute stroke.

Regarding this search for an effective treatment strategy, from a macroviewpoint it will be particularly important to find out "what should be done, and when should it be done?" Originally we did not think that the conduct of rTMS intervention for the treatment of upper extremity paralysis in acute stroke should be accorded so much importance. However, different from rTMS in the chronic phase of stroke, it is especially important to follow an order of priority when applying rTMS in acute stroke. Having an effective weapon such as rTMS it makes no sense to use up this method for a weak enemy, or to lose against a strong enemy that might have been defeated if one had applied rTMS. Currently, rTMS is still at the stage where it needs to be confirmed for which kind of cerebral symptoms it is effective. However, at the same time the question in which order rTMS should be applied is also of great importance in clinical practice.

Also from a microviewpoint there is still a mountain of problems; however, the determination of the optimal stimulation site, which is also still an unresolved issue of rTMS in the chronic phase of stroke, is particularly important because it is highly likely that it changes over time in acute stroke. At present the most widely used method for determining stimulation sites for the treatment of motor paralysis, regardless of whether it is for acute stroke or the chronic phase of stroke, is the detection of motor response by single-pulse TMS. However, it will be necessary to identify stimulation sites in accordance with, for instance, Penfield's homunculus or the Brodmann areas, and also to compare the effectiveness of the stimulation of "anatomically correct" sites such as stimulation sites that were determined based on functional brain imaging such as fMRI. A navigation system is required when conducting rTMS at such sites. With such a system it should be possible to conduct exactly localized stimulation by entering the targeted brain MRI data into a computer and through three-dimensional analysis of the direction of the coil and head.

Conclusions

Although it is tempting to draw attention to the effectiveness of rTMS as a new therapeutic intervention measure in acute stroke, the information that is available to date is still not sufficient. The most important point when applying rTMS in acute stroke is that the improvement that is achieved by rTMS intervention may not be inferior to the degree of recovery that would have been achieved with conventional intervention alone. It is necessary to carefully proceed with research being aware of the fact that the duration of the acute stage of stroke is limited and cannot be turned back.

References

1. Khedr EM, Ahmed MA, Fathy N, Rothwell JC. Therapeutic trial of repetitive transcranial magnetic stimulation after acute ischemic stroke. Neurology. 2005;65(3):466–8.
2. Liepert J, Zittel S, Weiller C. Improvement of dexterity by single session low-frequency repetitive transcranial magnetic stimulation over the contralesional motor cortex in acute stroke: a double-blind placebo-controlled crossover trial. Restor Neurol Neurosci. 2007;25(5–6):461–5.
3. Di Lazzaro V, Pilato F, Dileone M, Profice P, Capone F, Ranieri F, Musumeci G, Cianfoni A, Pasqualetti P, Tonali PA. Modulating cortical excitability in acute stroke: a repetitive TMS study. Clin Neurophysiol. 2008;119(3):715–23.
4. Khedr EM, Abdel-Fadeil MR, Farghali A, Qaid M. Role of 1 and 3 Hz repetitive transcranial magnetic stimulation on motor function recovery after acute ischaemic stroke. Eur J Neurol. 2009;16(12):1323–30.

5. Khedr EM, Etraby AE, Hemeda M, Nasef AM, Razek AA. Long-term effect of repetitive transcranial magnetic stimulation on motor function recovery after acute ischemic stroke. Acta Neurol Scand. 2010;121(1):30–7.
6. Khedr EM, Abo-Elfetoh N. Therapeutic role of rTMS on recovery of dysphagia in patients with lateral medullary syndrome and brainstem infarction. J Neurol Neurosurg Psychiatry. 2010;81(5):495–9.
7. Khaleel SH, Bayoumy IM, El-Nabil LM, Moustafa RR. Differential hemodynamic response to repetitive transcranial magnetic stimulation in acute stroke patients with cortical versus subcortical infarcts. Eur Neurol. 2010;63(6):337–42.
8. Chang WH, Kim YH, Bang OY, Kim ST, Park YH, Lee PK. Long-term effects of rTMS on motor recovery in patients after subacute stroke. J Rehabil Med. 2010;42(8):758–64.
9. Hsu YF, Huang YZ, Lin YY, Tang CW, Liao KK, Lee PL, Tsai YA, Cheng HL, Cheng H, Chern CM, Lee IH. Intermittent theta burst stimulation over ipsilesional primary motor cortex of subacute ischemic stroke patients: a pilot study. Brain Stimul. 2013;6(2):166–74.
10. Sasaki N, Mizutani S, Kakuda W, Abo M. Comparison of the effects of high- and low-frequency repetitive transcranial magnetic stimulation on upper limb hemiparesis in the early phase of stroke. J Stroke Cerebrovasc Dis. 2013;22(4):413–8.
11. Kim BR, Chun MH, Kim DY, Lee SJ. Effect of high- and low-frequency repetitive transcranial magnetic stimulation on visuospatial neglect in patients with acute stroke: a double-blind, sham-controlled trial. Arch Phys Med Rehabil. 2013;94(5):803–7.
12. Kim WS, Jung SH, Oh MK, Min YS, Lim JY, Paik NJ. Effect of repetitive transcranial magnetic stimulation over the cerebellum on patients with ataxia after posterior circulation stroke: a pilot study. J Rehabil Med. 2014;46(5):418–23.
13. Sasaki N, Kakuda W, Abo M. Bilateral high- and low-frequency rTMS in acute stroke patients with hemiparesis: a comparative study with unilateral high-frequency rTMS. Brain Inj. 2014;20:1–5.
14. Arboix A, Comes E, Massons J, García L, Oliveres M. Relevance of early seizures for in-hospital mortality in acute cerebrovascular disease. Neurology. 1996;47(6):1429–35.
15. Stinear C, Ackerley S, Byblow W. Rehabilitation is initiated early after stroke, but most motor rehabilitation trials are not: a systematic review. Stroke. 2013;44(7):2039–45.
16. Hsu WY, Cheng CH, Liao KK, Lee IH, Lin YY. Effects of repetitive transcranial magnetic stimulation on motor functions in patients with stroke: a meta-analysis. Stroke. 2012;43:1849–57.
17. Kakuda W, Abo M, Shimizu M, Sasanuma J, Okamoto T, Yokoi A, Taguchi K, Mitani S, Harashima H, Urushidani N, Urashima M, NEURO Investigators. A multi-center study on low-frequency rTMS combined with intensive occupational therapy for upper limb hemiparesis in post-stroke patients. J Neuroeng Rehabil. 2012;9(1):4.
18. Butler AJ, Wolf SL. Putting the brain on the map: use of transcranial magnetic stimulation to assess and induce cortical plasticity of upper-extremity movement. Phys Ther. 2007;87(6):719–36.
19. Marshall RS, Perera GM, Lazar RM, Krakauer JW, Constantine RC, DeLaPaz RL. Evolution of cortical activation during recovery from corticospinal tract infarction. Stroke. 2000;31:656–61.
20. Takeuchi N, Tada T, Toshima M, Matsuo Y, Ikoma K. Repetitive transcranial magnetic stimulation over bilateral hemispheres enhances motor function and training effect of paretic hand in patients after stroke. J Rehabil Med. 2009;41(13):1049–54.
21. Gao F, Wang S, Guo Y, Wang J, Lou M, Wu J, Ding M, Tian M, Zhang H. Protective effects of repetitive transcranial magnetic stimulation in a rat model of transient cerebral ischaemia: a microPET study. Eur J Nucl Med Mol Imaging. 2010;37:954–61.

Chapter 7
Case Presentation (Including TMS Device Handling Instructions)

Handling the TMS Device (MagPro)

Not many different types of TMS device are widely used in Japan. The MagPro manufactured by MagVenture (headquartered in Denmark) and the Magstim Rapid manufactured by Magstim (headquartered in the UK) seem to be the mainstream products (Fig. 7.1).

This section briefly describes how to actually handle MagVenture's MagPro, which is the device we use. When applying rTMS therapeutically, it is advisable to prepare a wheelchair with a head-holder cushion as shown in Fig. 7.2, as it is important to fix the position of the patient's head. It also goes without saying that it is essential to obtain the approval of the ethics committee of each institution when carrying out rTMS (rTMS is not approved for therapeutic purpose).

Starting Up the Device and Preparing the Patient

(i) After confirming that the patient is not in poor physical condition, seat the patient in a wheelchair as shown in Fig. 7.3. Then, tell the patient to relax, keeping his or her eyes closed (leaning against the wheelchair, with the back of his or her head in close contact with the head-holding cushion). Have the patient rest both hands and upper limbs on top of his or her thighs. Ensure the patient is not wearing spectacles or a wristwatch or carrying a mobile phone or cards that may be affected by a magnetic force when performing rTMS.

(ii) After connecting the figure-8 coil (manufactured by MagVenture) to the TMS device main unit, turn on the switch at the rear of the main unit. The LCD panel will start up after 20–30 seconds (Fig. 7.4).

(iii) If a cooler system is also fitted, ensure that the power supply to the system is also plugged in (if a cooler system is fitted, the coil surface is less likely to overheat, enabling continuous rTMS).

M. Abo, W. Kakuda, *Rehabilitation with rTMS*,
DOI 10.1007/978-3-319-20982-1_7

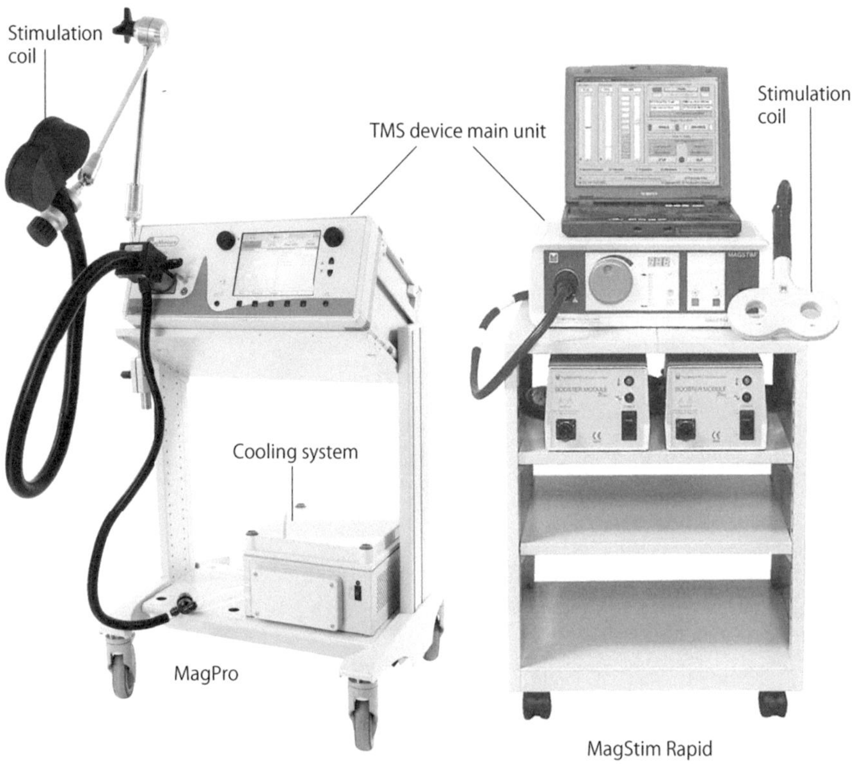

Fig. 7.1 Typical TMS device. The MagPro R30 shown in the photo also has a cooling system to prevent coil overheating

Determining the Stimulation Site and Intensity

(i) Insert the electromyography (EMG) line into the rear of the TMS device (the other end of the line is connected to the electrodes placed on the skin). Then, press the button under "Configure" displayed in the LCD panel (Fig. 7.4), and press the button under "MEP" (motor invoked potential) on the LCD panel, which is displayed next. As a result, the panel is now in EMG mode. Then, by moving the cursor up and down, set "Time Base" in EMG mode to "5 ms/div" (1 memory will be 5 ms and MEP occurring 20–25 ms after stimulation will be shown in the middle of the screen) and "Sensitivity" to "100 or 200 μV/div" (Fig. 7.5). Then, when you press button 1 (Fig. 7.4), "Status" at the top left of the panel will change from "Disabled (Red Screen)" to "Enabled (Green Screen)" and magnetic stimulation is enabled.

(ii) If applying rTMS in poststroke patients with upper limb hemiparesis, it is usual to apply rTMS in the hand and finger area of the primary motor cortex.

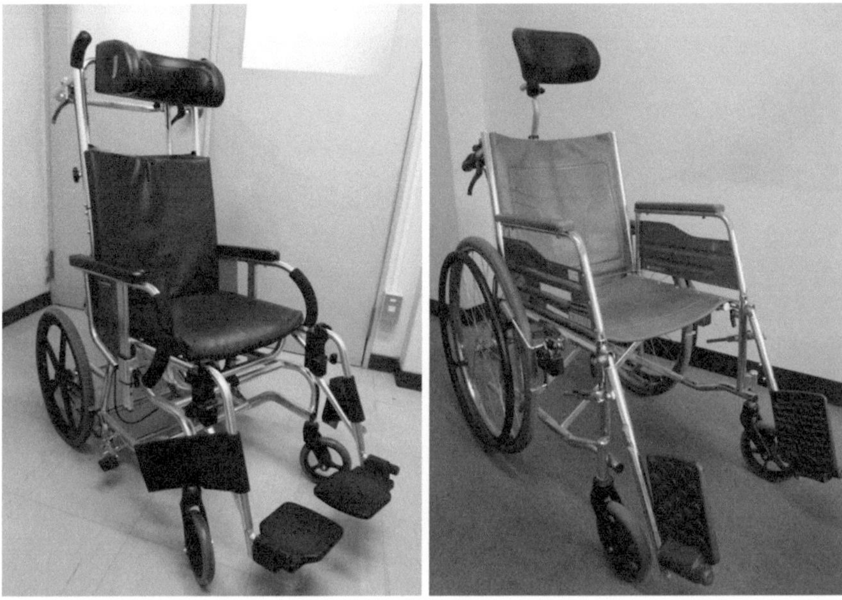

Fig. 7.2 Wheelchair with head-holder cushion. Designed so that the position of the head can be fixed during rTMS procedure

Fig. 7.3 Posture of patient during rTMS delivery. Sitting, relaxed with eyes closed

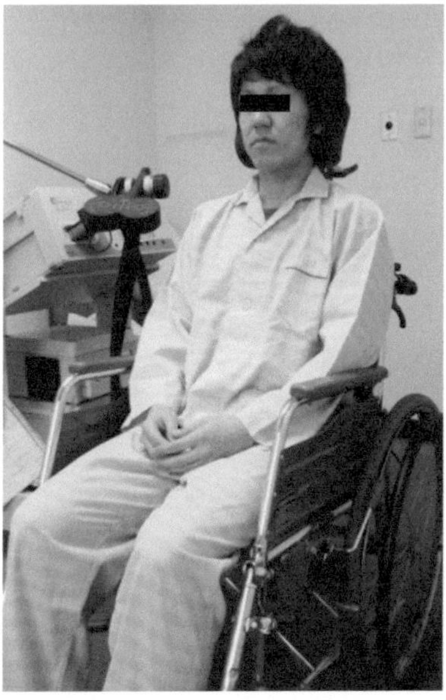

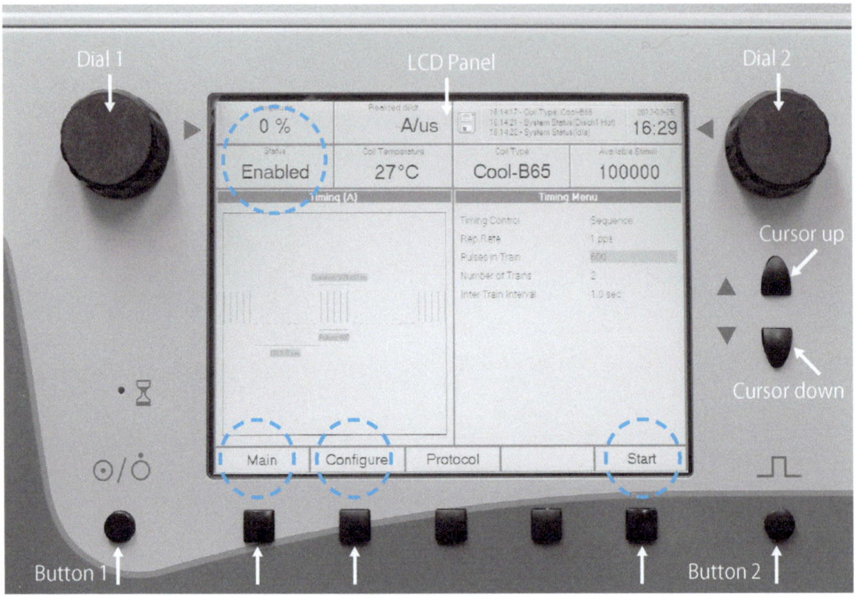

Fig. 7.4 LCD panel. All operations including confirmation of MEP waveform and setting of rTMS stimulation modality can be performed on this screen

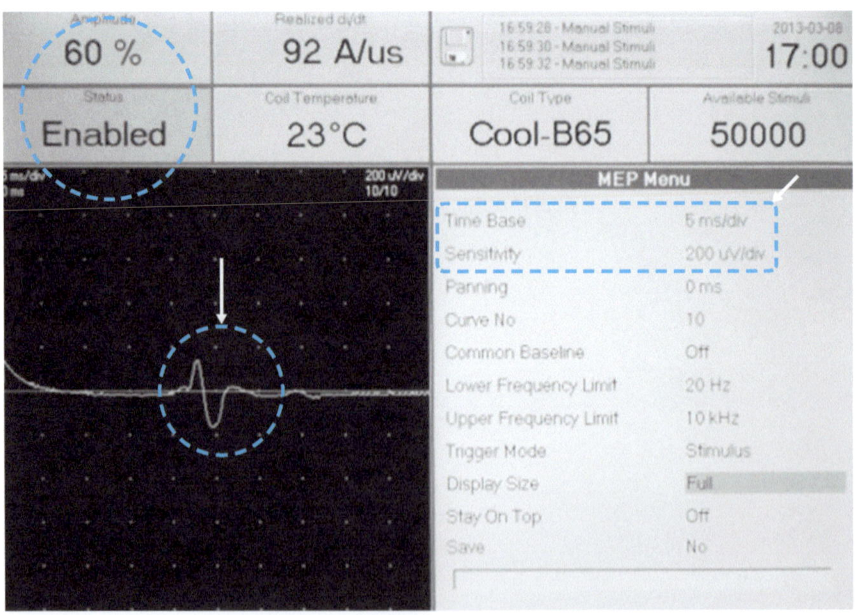

Fig. 7.5 MEP waveform. By applying single pulse magnetic stimulation to the primary motor cortex, it is possible to induce MEP from the muscles at the stimulation site

Our practice is to take the primary motor cortex corresponding to the first dorsal interosseous muscle (FDI muscle) of the nonparalyzed upper limb in the nonlesional hemisphere as the stimulation site for low-frequency rTMS. Therefore, when determining the stimulation site for upper limb hemiparesis, first attach the electrodes of the surface EMG to the FDI muscle of the nonparalyzed upper limb as shown in Fig. 7.6 [In the figure, the red (b) and black (c) plugs are the measurement electrodes, and the green (a) plug is the earth.]

(iii) The person delivering rTMS places the figure-8 coil near the primary motor cortex on the unaffected hemisphere, presses button 2 (Fig. 7.4) or the button for single pulse stimulation next to the coil, and, while repeating magnetic stimulation in single pulses, gradually increases the stimulation intensity (Fig. 7.7). Stimulation intensity can be increased by turning dial 1 (Fig. 7.4) clockwise [stimulation intensity is shown in percent (%) as "Amplitude"]. In the case of MagPro, it is better to start from an intensity of approximately 20 % and, after applying around approximately 3–4 pulses of stimulation each time, increasing stimulation intensity in increments of 3–5 %. Then, detect the site at which movement of the nonparalyzed index finger can be induced most noticeably, moving the site of application of the figure-8 coil bit by bit. It is better to visually confirm movement of the index finger initially and then to check that MEP of the FDI muscle of the nonparalyzed upper limb is being induced on the EMG (Fig. 7.5).

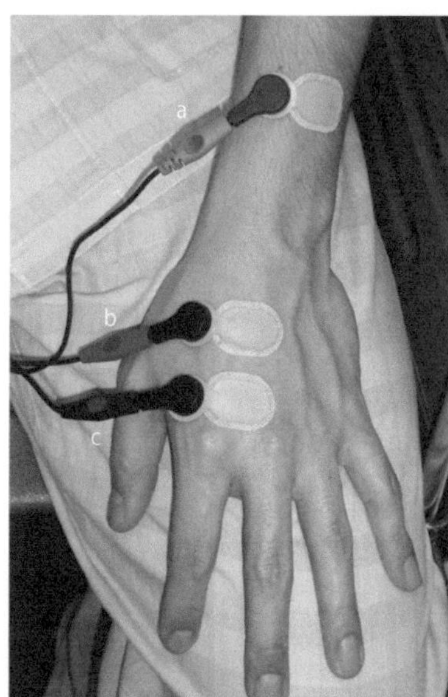

Fig. 7.6 Attachment of the EMG electrodes. Electrodes are often attached to the FDI muscle, but can also be attached to the abductor pollicis muscle

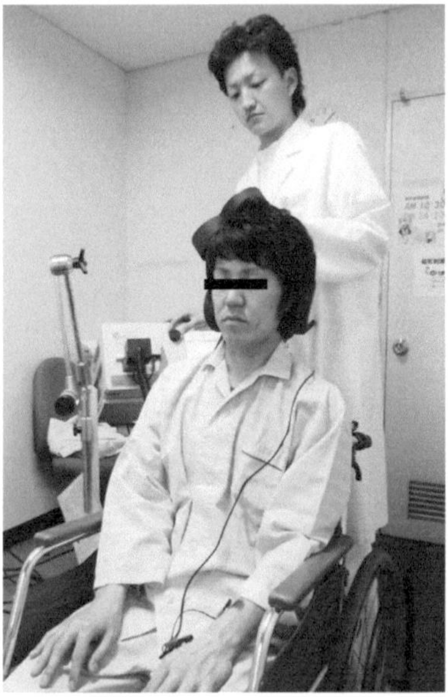

Fig. 7.7 Confirmation of the stimulation site. Detect the site at which MEP can be induced most noticeably, gradually increasing the stimulation intensity by turning the dial of the main unit with your right hand

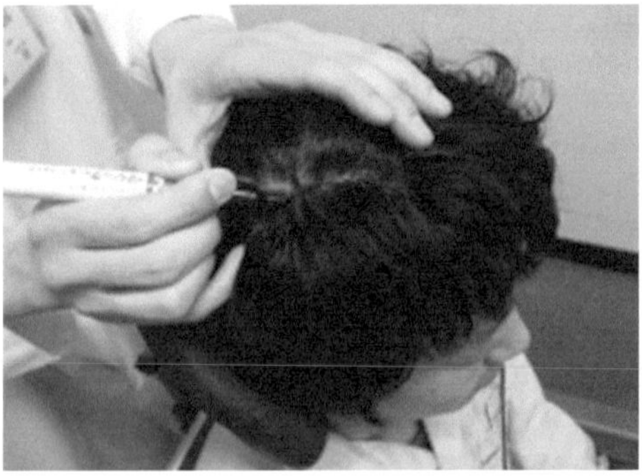

Fig. 7.8 Marking of stimulation site. Mark the stimulation site to prevent displacement of the stimulation site in subsequent rTMS sessions

(iv) Once the site at which MEP can be induced most noticeably is determined, measure the resting motor threshold, which is defined as "the minimum stimulation intensity at which MEP with amplitude of 50 μV or more can be induced with a probability of 50 % of more." Then, take 90 % of this intensity as the rTMS stimulation intensity (e.g., if the resting motor threshold is 60 %, the stimulation intensity used in therapy will be 54 %. Then, movement of the nonparalyzed hand should not occur during the rTMS treatment).

(v) Once the stimulation site is determined, upon obtaining the patient's approval, mark the stimulation site with a marker pen as shown in Fig. 7.8 to ensure that the site does not move in subsequent rTMS sessions. While it is, of course, advisable to confirm the stimulation site by inducing MEP each time rTMS is

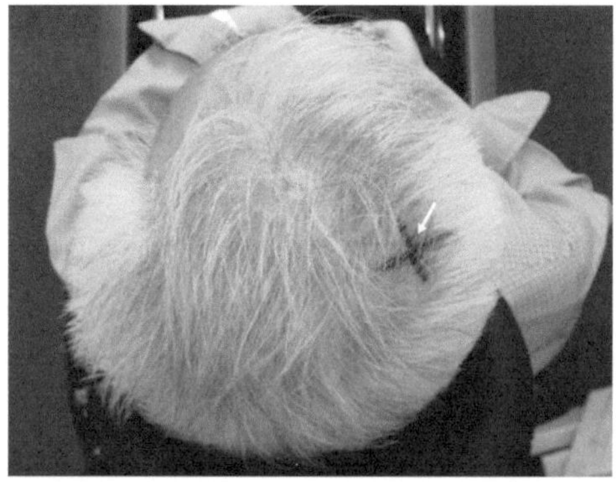

Fig. 7.9 Example of marked stimulation site. It is advisable to draw a cross with a marker pen

delivered, marking the approximate stimulation site in this way will facilitate determination of the stimulation site on subsequent occasions. Figure 7.9 shows an example in which the marked site is seen from directly above. The hand and finger area of the primary motor cortex is often situated approximately 2–5 finger breadths away from and slightly in front of Cz (vertex) based on the International 10–20 Method for EEG.

(vi) If movement of the hand of the nonparalyzed upper limb is not induced even after the stimulation intensity is increased to approximately 90 %, it is possible that the coil is improperly positioned, but, in some patients, movement cannot be induced even when stimulation intensity is 100 %. This is presumably due to the thickness of the skull. In such cases, it is better to lower the motor threshold and create a situation in which movement of the hand will be induced more easily by extending and elevating the nonparalyzed upper limb and dorsiflexing the wrist. This will make it more difficult to reliably set the exact stimulation intensity but will probably make it easier to determine the stimulation site.

(vii) If applying high-frequency rTMS to the primary motor cortex in the unaffected hemisphere in poststroke patients with paralyzed upper limb, first attach the EMG to the FDI muscle of the paralyzed upper limb. Then, detect the site at which movement of the paralyzed FDI muscle can be induced and the site at which MEP of the paralyzed FDI muscle can be induced by stimulating the primary motor cortex of the affected hemisphere. However, it is not uncommon for it to be impossible to invoke or induce movement and MEP of the paralyzed FDI muscle even at maximum stimulation intensity. In such cases, it is probably better to first detect the site at which movement and MEP of the nonparalyzed FDI muscle can be invoked or induced and then determine the corresponding site as the rTMS application site.

(viii) The right or left inferior frontal gyrus of frontal lobe is reportedly often selected as the rTMS application site in poststroke aphasic patients. While it is normally advisable to use an MRI navigation system to determine the position of the inferior frontal gyrus, only a limited number of institutions have such a system. However, areas F7 and F8 according to the International 10–20

Method have been confirmed to correspond to the left and right inferior frontal gyrus respectively. Therefore, therapeutic rTMS in aphasic patients (especially patients with motor aphasia) is probably actually applied in this F7 area or F8 area based on the International 10–20 Method. The stimulation intensity of rTMS in patients with aphasia is usually determined by measuring the resting motor threshold of the nonparalyzed upper limb FDI muscle in the same way as for upper limb hemiparesis and setting intensity at about 90 % of this.

Application of rTMS

(i) If applying TMS in the form of therapeutic rTMS, first set the "Waveform" and "Timing Menu" (Fig. 7.10). The nature of rTMS stimulation (stimulation modality) will be determined based mainly on the Timing Menu.

(ii) With the Main Menu displayed on the right side of the panel, move the cursor to Waveform and select "Biphasic" (not Monophasic) (Fig. 7.11). Since the magnetic energy released from the coil is greater with "biphasic" than with "monophasic," it is better to use "biphasic" if using rTMS therapeutically.

(iii) When you press the button under "Main" on the LCD panel (Fig. 7.4), the word "Timing" will appear, and the "Timing Menu" will be displayed on the right side of the panel. Then set the stimulation modality. "Rep Rate (repetitive rate)" shown here denotes frequency (pps = pulses per second), and "Pulses in Train" denotes the number of pulses delivered in one stimulation train. "Number of Trains" shows how many stimulation trains are to be administered overall, and "Inter Train Interval" shows the interval between trains.

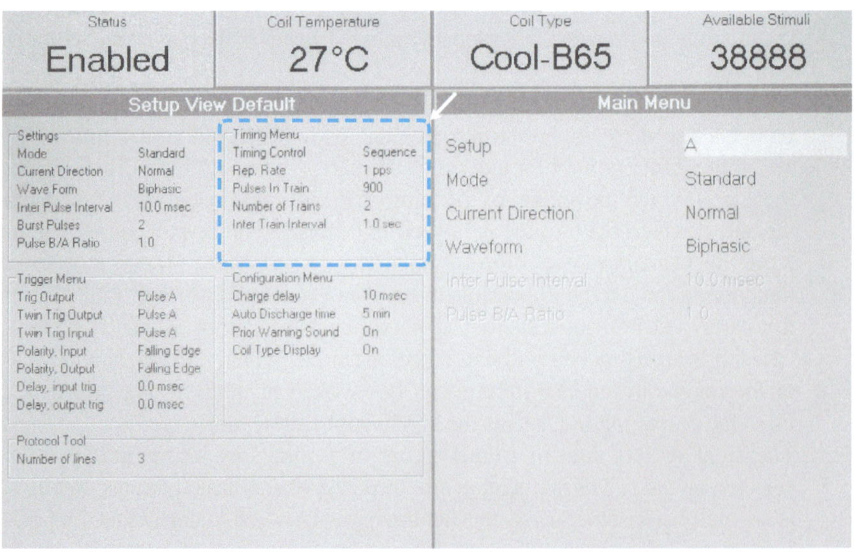

Fig. 7.10 Timing Menu display. Stimulation modality (nature of stimulation) is displayed in the form of Timing Menu

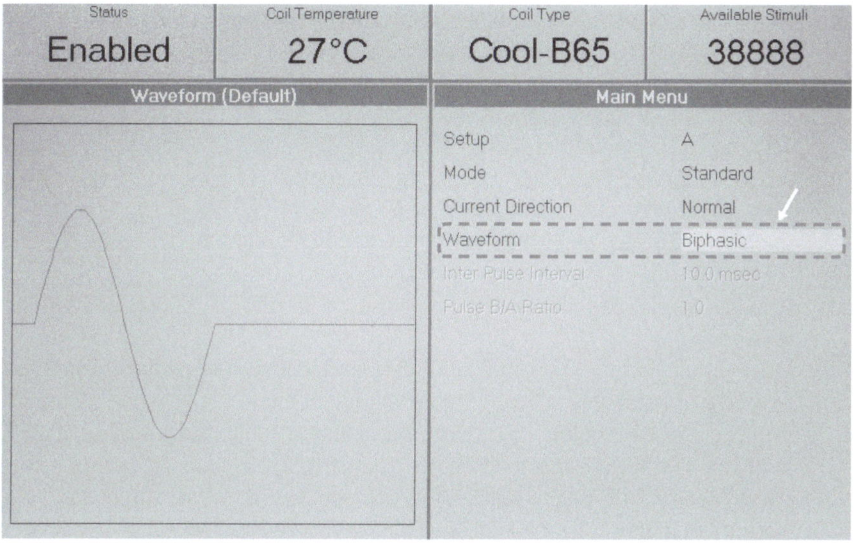

Fig. 7.11 Selection of stimulation waveform. Biphasic waveform is advisable if using as rTMS for therapeutic purposes

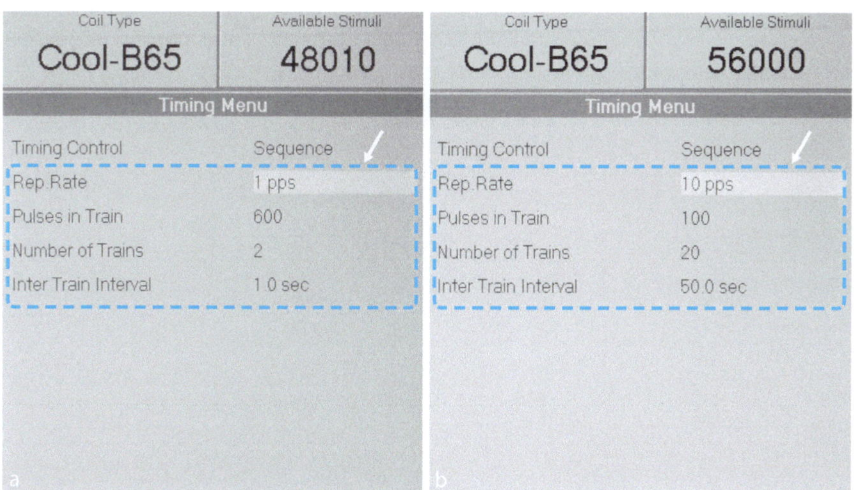

Fig. 7.12 Commonly used settings for low-frequency and high-frequency rTMS. (**a**) Setting for low-frequency rTMS (1 Hz). (**b**) Setting for high-frequency rTMS (10 Hz)

(iv) If delivering low-frequency (1 Hz) rTMS for 20 minutes, set as shown in Fig. 7.12a. First, set Rep Rate as 1 pps (1 Hz) and Pulses in Train as 600. This means that 600 pulses at 1 Hz will be delivered per train; in other words, 10 minutes of 1 Hz stimulation will be delivered. If you then set the Inter Train Interval at 1 second and the Number of Trains at 2, this means in effect that 2 stimulation trains (in other words, 600 pulses × 2 trains = 1200 pulses) will be delivered continuously, lasting 20 minutes.

(v) To deliver high-frequency (10 Hz) rTMS using 10 second pulses at 50 second intervals for 20 minutes, set as shown in Fig. 7.12b. First, set the Rep Rate as 10 pps (10 Hz) and Pulses in Train as 100 (100 pulses at 10 Hz per train = 10 seconds) and the Inter Train Interval at 50 seconds. This means that one train lasts a total of 1 minute comprised of 10 seconds of 10 Hz stimulation and an interval of 50 seconds. Moreover if you set the Number of Trains as 20, this means that this stimulation train will be repeated 20 times, lasting 20 minutes. In other words, this means that 100 pulses × 20 trains = 2000 pulses will be delivered.

(vi) Once you have finished setting stimulation modality, use the fixed arm fitted to the TMS main unit to firmly fix the stimulation coil to the marked stimulation site as shown in Fig. 7.13. Next, press button 1 (Fig. 7.4) to turn "Status" at the top left of the panel to "Enabled" (Green). Then, press the button below "Start" on the LCD panel (Fig. 7.4). When you do this, the set stimulation will start immediately.

(vii) During rTMS delivery, you will be accompanied by a doctor, as a general rule, in case an adverse effect or adverse event occurs. rTMS is painless, and patients we have actually treated have never complained about clearly localized head pain. However, when the stimulation intensity increases, the muscle surrounding the stimulation site is directly stimulated, and muscle contraction of the temporal region, palpebral part, buccal region, etc. may occur at the same time as the stimulation. In addition, in patients with noticeable body

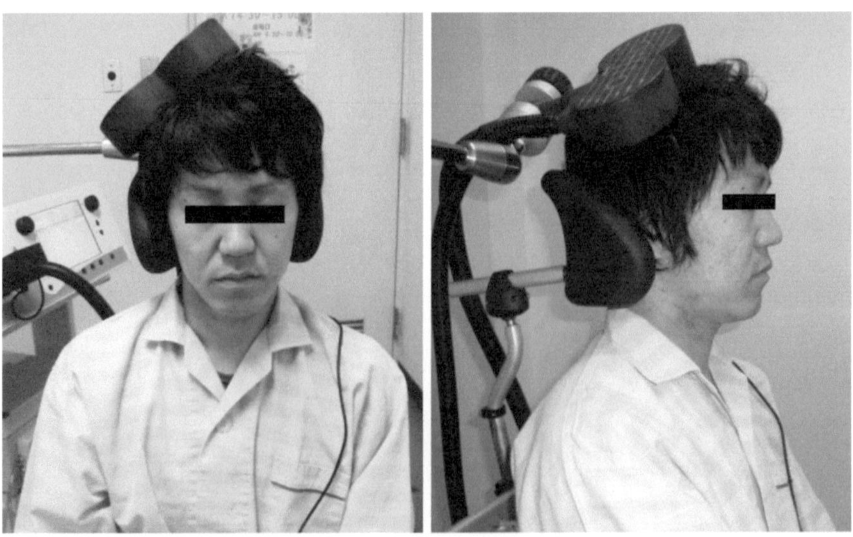

Fig. 7.13 Actual rTMS delivery. The stimulation coil is held by a rigid arm

movements (patients who find it difficult to maintain the same posture), since it is not uncommon for the coil to become displaced, ensure that stimulation is applied to the right site by checking the position of the coil as required and correcting the position of the coil if necessary.

Case 1

A 75-year-old male patient for whom importance was attached to ADL guidance in occupational therapy as part of NEURO-15 and an improvement of motor function in a paralyzed upper limb was linked to ADL.

Medical History and Background

In October 2010 (at the age of 74), the right-handed patient was taken to a nearby hospital by ambulance after weakness occurred on the left side of his body. He was diagnosed with right putaminal hemorrhage and admitted to hospital as an emergency. After being treated with conservative therapy, he was transferred to a convalescent rehabilitation hospital in December 2010. For approximately 3 months after admission, the patient underwent rehabilitation, but left upper limb hemiparesis persisted, and it was difficult for the patient to use his left upper limb practically. In February 2012, the patient was admitted to our hospital for treatment of the left upper limb hemiparesis. Before being admitted to the hospital, the patient went to day care four times a week. The patient lived with his wife and other family members and had worked as a carpenter for approximately 60 years before the onset of symptoms.

Pretreatment Physical Findings

[General physical findings] Height 165 cm, weight 50 kg

[Consciousness] Clear

[Higher brain function] Mini Mental State Examination (MMSE) 27/30 points. Otherwise, satisfactory

[Motor system] Evidence of left upper limb hemiparesis. Compensatory movement with trunk lateral flexion/rotation was observed during flexion of the shoulder joint, and poor dynamic stability of proximal portion was found. Brunnstrom recovery stage (BRS) was equal to stage III for left upper limb and stage IV for left hand and finger. In the flexor muscles of the left upper limb, a clear increase in muscle tone was found, and an increase in the biceps tendon and brachioradialis reflex of the left upper limb was also found.

[Sensory system] Superficial sensation and deep sensation of the left upper limb are both at a moderately dull level.

[Standing and walking] Patient is stable when standing and can move by walking independently within his own home. However, outside, the patient uses a T-shaped cane and needs monitoring. He does not use an orthosis.

[ADL] The patient is independent except when taking a bath. He hardly uses his left upper limb in ADL. When he goes out, he goes with his wife.

Evaluation Results

The results of each evaluation performed from the time of admission to 4 weeks after discharge are as shown in Table 7.1.

Pretreatment Image Findings

A high-intensity area indicating old cerebral hemorrhage in the right putamen was found in head MRI (T2-weighted image).

Table 7.1 Evaluation results

Evaluation method/items		At admission	At discharge	4 weeks after discharge
BRS[a]	Left upper limb	III	III	III
	Left hand and finger	IV	IV	IV
MAS[b]	Left elbow flexor muscles	1	1	1
	Left wrist flexors	1	1	1
	Left finger flexor muscles	1	1	1
ROM[c] (passive)	Left shoulder joint flexion	90	100	140
	Left shoulder joint abduction	90	100	140
FMA (upper limb)[d]	Overall score	43	47	16
WMFT[e]	15 tasks perf. time (seconds)	172.83	83.99	82.38
	FAS[f]	45	53	50
10-second test (grip and release) (times)		3	6	6

[a]BRS (Brunnstrom recovery stage)
[b]MAS (modified Ashworth scale)
[c]ROM (range of motion)
[d]FMA (Fugl-Meyer assessment)
[e]WMFT (Wolf motor function test)
[f]FAS (functional ability scale)

Patient's Needs, Treatment Goal, and Treatment Plan

The need of the patient was for "the left arm and hand and finger to be completely returned to normal." However, there was a severe degree of upper limb hemiparesis, and practical use was judged difficult. We, therefore, focused on the hand and finger with comparatively good function and, upon consultation with the patient himself, set a concrete treatment goal of "being able to hold a plastic bottle or can." In addition, since the left upper limb was hardly used in ADL, we added the objective of "increasing opportunities to use the left upper limb in ADL." Based on this, we adopted the hospital treatment plan of providing OT focusing on training to improve the dynamic stability of the left shoulder joint and left hand and finger holding training, while delivering rTMS to the hand and finger area of the primary motor cortex in the nonlesional hemisphere on a daily basis.

Content of Rehabilitation Program

(i) Application of low-frequency rTMS to the hand and finger area of the primary motor cortex in the left (nonlesional) hemisphere (20 minutes twice daily)
(ii) Range of motion (ROM) training aimed at increasing the ROM of the left shoulder joint
(iii) Stretching aimed at reducing the muscle tone of the left shoulder joint, elbow joint, wrist, and finger joints
(iv) Holding training and pinching training using various objects to improve left hand dexterity
(v) Facilitation training aimed at increasing voluntary movement of the triceps brachii muscle, extensor carpi radialis brevis muscle, extensor carpi ulnaris muscle, and extensor digitorum muscle of the upper limb using EMS (electric muscle stimulation)
(vi) Facilitation training for shoulder muscles aimed at increasing dynamic stability of the left upper limb proximal portion
(vii) Guidance on actively using the left upper limb in ADL in hospital (eating, getting changed, washing face, washing hair, etc.)
(viii) Self-exercise to improve function of left upper limb for 2 hours daily, guidance focusing on object holding and manipulation training

Course

From the day following admission to hospital, we delivered rehabilitation focusing on training to improve the dynamic stability of the left upper limb proximal portion and left hand holding training. We also provided due guidance on using the left upper limb in ADL. As a result, from around the fifth day in hospital, extension of the left elbow joint and palmar abduction using the left abductor pollicis muscle became possible, and the patient himself also began to say that he has more opportunities to use his left hand more than before. At discharge, shoulder joint ROM was also greater, and the patient could grip a plastic bottle or can and raise it to his mouth. As shown in Table 7.1, in evaluation, a noticeable improvement in WMFT was found. The patient himself also fully understood the need to complete the rehabilitation program and self-exercise and worked hard throughout. After discharge, he reportedly completed the independent training at home almost every day and, 4 weeks after discharge, the improvement in the motor function attained at discharge had been maintained.

Discussion

The patient had moderate hemiparesis of the left upper limb and left hand and finger and hardly used the left upper limb in ADL. We, therefore, focused on the hand and finger with comparatively good function and adopted the approach of focusing on improvement of hand function with the aim of making the left hand an assistive hand. Since the restricted ROM of the shoulder joint was also obstructing upper limb manipulation, we took the approach of improving the dynamic stability of the upper limb proximal portion in addition to improving the ROM of the shoulder joint. We believe that our approach of providing ADL guidance as required combined with improvement of function helped to increase frequency of use of the left upper limb and left hand in ADL. The patient himself commented that "I gradually became able to use my left hand in life on the ward," and our approach may also have helped to increase awareness of using the left upper limb in ADL and to increase training motivation.

Patient's Impressions

> After receiving the rTMS treatment, I am able to use my left hand, which had previously hardly used at all, and to understand how to use it. Since I received not only functional training but also guidance on how to use my left hand in daily life from the day after my admission, I was able to practice this gradually while in hospital and felt that I used my left hand more and more frequently day by day.

Conclusion

Alongside improvement in function, we provided the patient with guidance on using his left upper limb, which was previously unusable, in ADL and combined intensive OT with rTMS. As a result, the holding function of the hand and frequency of use of the left upper limb in ADL showed improvement both subjectively and objectively. This suggested that the approach of including ADL guidance using the paralyzed side in addition to rTMS treatment and functional training is a useful therapeutic intervention.

Case 2

A 65-year-old male patient whose handwriting movements became independent and who was able to return to work as a result of continuous rTMS on an outpatient basis after completion of NEURO-15.

Medical History and Background

In February 2010 (at the age of 64), the right-handed patient noticed heaviness in the head, difficulty articulating, and weakness on the right side of the body and, when examined at a nearby hospital, was diagnosed with cerebral infarction, urgently admitted, and underwent emergency treatment at the hospital. He was later transferred to another hospital for rehabilitation purposes, and although he was discharged after 5 months in hospital, he still had hemiparesis of the right upper and lower limbs. It was, therefore, judged difficult for him to return to work, and he retired for a time. However, the patient was admitted to our department in November 2010 because he wished to undergo specific rehabilitation for the right hemiplegia with the aim of returning to work. The patient had a history of hypertension and was taking antihypertension drugs, etc. He lived with his wife and second daughter. He previously commuted to his company by train. His hobby was golf, but he was no longer playing and spent his days helping with the housework and going for walks.

Pretreatment Physical Findings

[General physical findings] Height 165 cm, weight 65 kg. In a standing position, the center of gravity was offset to the nonparalyzed side, and the upper limb on the paralyzed side showed slight inner rotation of the shoulder joint and slight flexion of the elbow joint.

[Consciousness] Clear

[Higher brain function] The patient himself was aware of his difficulty articulating but had no problem communicating. The higher brain function screening test showed no other abnormal findings.

[Cranial nervous system] Evidence of dysphagia and facial paralysis on the right side

[Motor system] Moderate hemiplegia was found in the right upper limb. BRS on the paralyzed side was equal to stage IV for upper limb and stage IV for hand and finger, there were severe contractions of the flexor muscles, and an increase in reflexes was also observed.

[Sensory system] Superficial sensation and deep sensation are both normal. There is no sign of pain, sense of numbness, etc. on the paralyzed side.

[Standing and walking] The patient can walk independently indoors using an ankle-foot orthosis. However, outdoors, he uses a stick as he stumbles and is unstable. An increase in flexor muscle spasticity of the paralyzed upper limb was observed when walking.

[ADL] While the patient could perform basic movements and ADLs independently, frequency of use of the paralyzed upper limb was low, and use was restricted to certain actions such as wringing a cloth or towel, tearing off toilet paper, or fastening a belt. Although the patient had attempted performing chopstick and writing movements with the paralyzed upper limb, increased spasticity of the flexor muscles of the entire upper limb from the shoulder girdle through the hand made this virtually impossible.

Evaluation Results

The results of each evaluation performed from the time of admission to 8 weeks after discharge are as shown in Table 7.2.

Pretreatment Image Findings

A low-density area suggesting old infarction lesions in the left basilar pons was found in plain head CT.

Table 7.2 Evaluation results (Case 2)

Evaluation method/evaluation items		At admission	At discharge	8 weeks after discharge
MAS	Elbow flexor muscles	1^+	1	1
	Wrist flexor muscles	1^+	1	1
	Finger flexor muscles	1^+	0	0
FMA (upper limb)	Overall score	55	57	–
WMFT	15 tasks perf. time (seconds)	87.92	60.02	50.98
STEF[a]		27	45	–

[a]STEF (simple test for evaluating hand function)

Patient's Needs, Treatment Goal, and Treatment Plan

The needs of the patient were that he wanted to write with his right hand and wanted to eat holding chopsticks in his right hand. However, upon consultation with the patient, we set the treatment goals of being able to write his name with a pencil and being able to eat with a self-help device chopstick, since, in view of the existing status of isolated movements of the upper limb/hand and finger, work for a sustained period of time would be difficult and use of a self-help device was considered necessary. Based on this, we adopted the hospital treatment plan of delivering functional training aimed at facilitating isolated movements of the paralyzed upper limb proximal portion and hand and finger, and providing OT focusing on task-oriented ADL training such as handwriting and chopstick movements, while delivering low-frequency rTMS for 40 minutes on a daily basis throughout hospital stay.

Content of Rehabilitation Program

(i) Application of low-frequency (1 Hz) rTMS to the hand and finger area of the primary motor cortex in the right (nonlesional) hemisphere (40 minutes once daily)
(ii) Static stretch aimed at reducing muscle tone of flexor muscles from shoulder joint through finger joints (for approximately 1–2 minutes at the end of each movement session in individual OT; guidance to do self-stretching at the end of each task in self-exercise)
(iii) Repeated performance of single joint movements from shoulder joint through wrist joint (while applying resistance according to strength of patient's own muscle force output)
(iv) Repeated performance of multijoint movements from shoulder joint through wrist joint (especially aiming to achieve eccentric contraction of agonists during movements)
(v) Facilitation of isolated movements of hand and finger using objects (with awareness of grading of hand and finger control, from task of fixing object using chuck pinch to extending index finger only with object fixed using chuck pinch)
(vi) Self-exercise done focusing on program aimed at improving isolated movements (gross motor skills) and exercise endurance

Course

When we provided rehabilitation aimed at reducing hypertonia of the hand and finger for 3 days from the day of admission, a reduction in the muscle tone of the hand and finger began to be noticed from around the second day in hospital, and the patient was able to perform hand and finger movements multiple times. The patient himself also recognized that it had become easier to move his hand and finger.

After confirming that isolated movements of the hand had been facilitated, we focused on single-joint movements and multijoint movements on the paralyzed upper limb proximal side. However, though single-joint movements were possible, when it came to multijoint movements and composite movements, increased muscle tone of the wrist flexors and biceps brachii muscle and compensatory movements such as elevation of the shoulder blade and shoulder abduction were observed. We, therefore, provided rehabilitation consisting mainly of single-joint movements, with particular focus on the eccentric contraction of muscles prone to increased muscle tone. As a result, after 1 week in hospital, increased muscle tone and excessive effort in multijoint movements and composite movements were no longer evident, and the patient himself also said that he had "got the knack of relaxing."

At discharge, he achieved the handwriting movements he had hoped for, as expressed by himself that he was able to write characters more or less the same as before his stroke, and he was also able to perform face washing and drinking movements in everyday life. However, when it came to chopstick movements, while the patient started out well, he gradually became fatigued, and eventually his fingers would no longer work. Consequently, at the behest of the patient himself, it was decided that the patient would visit the outpatient rehabilitation clinic of the hospital once a week and undergo 20 minutes of low-frequency (1 Hz) rTMS and 40 minutes of individual rehabilitation.

In the outpatient rehabilitation, we continued to facilitate isolated movements of the hand and finger and also carried out OT focusing on improving endurance of the proximal side of the paralyzed upper limb. As a result, 2 months after starting outpatient rehabilitation, the patient became able to use chopsticks to the end of a meal. After 4 months, the outpatient rehabilitation came to end, partly at the request of the patient who had returned to work and was now busy with work.

Discussion

The patient presented moderate right hemiparesis, and it was considered that, functionally, the right hand was usable as an assistive hand. However, during movement, increased muscle tone of the paralyzed upper limb flexor muscles and excessive effort caused actual movement patterns to be clumsy. As a result, the patient hardly used the paralyzed upper limb in ADL, and we believe that learned nonuse and decrease in muscle function due to nonuse occurred. When we carried out NEURO-15 to address this situation, functional improvement of the paralyzed upper limb and increased frequency of use in ADL were observed as a result of intervention during hospitalization. We were able to link this to a return to work by continuing ongoing intervention through rehabilitation on an outpatient basis.

It has been suggested that NEURO-15 is also effective in reducing the spasticity of the paralyzed upper limb, and in this patient, this spasticity-reducing effect was indeed evident, and this may have led to the patient learning normal movements by controlling excessive effort and compensatory movements. On this occasion, the effect of NEURO-15 was most evident after 1 week in hospital, and we believe we were able to prevent an increase in spasticity and facilitate the learning of normal movements through the grading intensive OT treatment content in line with this effect.

For this patient, we continued regularly delivering rTMS treatment on an outpatient basis after completion of NEURO-15. In the case of patients like this patient who have no particular problem visiting hospital, the strategy of continuing rTMS on an outpatient basis may be useful.

In the case of this patient, we began rTMS treatment before 1 year had elapsed from onset because the time he planned to return to work was approaching. Eligibility criteria for NEURO-15 as of December 2012 state that the time from symptom onset to therapy must be at least 1 year, and previously, in almost all patients, we delivered rTMS treatment once 1 year had elapsed from onset. However, safety of staring treatment from the acute phase has also been confirmed in many papers, and, in the future, we will examine the usefulness of introduction of rTMS treatment at an earlier stage.

Patient Impressions

> I am now able to write. The fact that I am now able to write better (with my right hand) than with my left hand is like a dream. I now intend to continue practicing so I can use chopsticks a little better.

Conclusion

In this patient, we were able to achieve the objectives of chopstick and handwriting movements by carrying out NEURO-15 based on consideration of reduction of spasticity and self-control of muscle force output. Achievement of the target movements also produced motivation to achieve other ADL movements and return to work, and we were able to help the patient to achieve a more independent lifestyle.

Case 3

A 70-year-old female patient for whom further improvement in upper limb motor function on the paralyzed side was observed as a result of repeated NEURO-15.

Medical History and Background

In April 2001 (at the age of 60), the right-handed patient developed intracerebral hemorrhage (left thalamus) and was urgently admitted to a nearby hospital. She was later hospitalized in a convalescent rehabilitation hospital for approximately 6 months. Following long-term rehabilitation for right hemiparesis, her right upper limb improved to the level of an assistive hand, and she was discharged. However, the patient soon developed depression, preventing rehabilitation for right hemiparesis, and contracture of the right elbow and wrist joint became evident. She was then admitted to a psychiatric hospital for approximately 1 year for treatment of depression.

In May 2011, the patient was admitted to our hospital for the purpose of intensive rehabilitation for right upper limb hemiparesis (first time). As a result of NEURO-15, right upper limb motor function improved, and the patient regained eating movements using a chopsticks-type self-help device. Following discharge, the patient was even able to attempt horse riding, which was her hobby, while undergoing treatment such as ambulatory rehabilitation, swimming, electric therapy, and acupuncture. However, in September 2012, she was once again hospitalized in our hospital for further intensive rehabilitation for right upper limb hemiparesis (second time). The patient had a history of hypertension and hyperlipidemia and was still on medication (antithrombotics, antihypertensives, vasodilators, lipid-lowering agents, etc.). She had been working in the teaching profession until the age of 50, had then become a full-time housewife, and now lived alone.

Pretreatment Physical Findings (Second Time)

[General physical findings] Height 138 cm, weight 44 kg. Right scapula is depressed, right upper limb as a whole tends to internally rotate, and subluxation of approximately one fingerbreadth is evident. The trunk bends to the right, and there is a tendency for a round back. The neck was extended to hold the head horizontal from round back, and muscles from neck to trapezius were overstrained.

[Consciousness] Clear

[Higher brain function] No abnormal observations (Results of evaluation do not show depression.)

[Cranial nervous system] No abnormal observations

[Motor system] Right upper limb shows paresis and is at level of assistive hand. Although there is contraction of the MP joint and PIP joint of the ring finger on the right hand, hand BRS is equal to stage IV. Increased muscle tone of flexor muscles was observed in right wrist and all finger joints. Upper limb BRS is equal to stage III, and increased muscle tone was observed in flexor muscles of right elbow joint. During right upper limb manipulation, motor ataxia as a result of difficulty adjusting the muscle output force of the agonist and antagonist muscles was observed.

[Sensory system] Surface sensation and deep sensation are both slightly dull on the left side of the body and in particular very dull in the hand. Numbness was observed in the right side of the body.

[Standing and walking] Indoors, the patient walks independently, and outdoors she is independent walking with a stick.

[ADL] Although she was independent in all ADL, she was unable to do housework movements herself and asked a helper to do them. She moved around the neighborhood by electric bicycle.

Evaluation Results

The results of each evaluation performed at admission and at discharge the first and second times were as shown in Table 7.3.

Pretreatment Image Findings

Abnormal signal intensity indicating old hemorrhagic lesion was observed in the left thalamus in head MRI (T2-weighted image).

Patient's Needs, Treatment Goal, and Treatment Plan

The patient's need during the hospitalization for the first time was "to eat with chopsticks," and, at the time of discharge, she was able to achieve this activity using a chopstick-type self-help device. During the hospitalization for the second time, her need was "to ride a horse, holding the reins in here right hand and the whip in her

Table 7.3 Evaluation results (Case 3)

Evaluation method/items		First time		Second time	
		At admission	At discharge	At admission	At discharge
BRS	Right upper limb	III	IV	III	V
	Right hand finger	IV	IV	IV	IV
MAS	Wrist flexor muscles	1	0	1	0
	Finger flexor muscles	4	4	3	1^+
FMA (upper limb)	Overall score	45	51	50	53
WMFT	15 tasks perf. time (seconds)	579.79	567.8	485.09	229.04
	FAS	37	40	44	49

left," and we set this as the treatment goal. Based on this, we adopted the hospital treatment plan of providing OT focusing on reducing contracture and spasticity of the finger joints and increasing sensory function of the hand finger, while delivering low-frequency rTMS to the hand finger area of the primary motor cortex in the unaffected hemisphere on a daily basis.

Content of Rehabilitation Program (at Admission for the Second Time)

(i) Low-frequency (1 Hz) rTMS to the hand finger area of the primary motor cortex in the right (nonlesional) hemisphere (40 minutes once daily)
(ii) Stretching aimed at reducing the muscle tone of the elbow joint and finger joints and reducing contracture of the right ring finger (focusing on any increased muscle tone observed during self- training)
(iii) Facilitation of right wrist dorsiflexion and right finger joint extension for holding reins
(iv) Mobilization and facilitation training of the trunk, neck, and scapular muscles for adjustment of the alignment of the trunk and scapula (including improvement of the subluxation)
(v) Facilitation of flexion of right finger joints and sensory re-education training for surface and deep sensation for gripping and holding reins
(vi) Similar movement training for gripping and manipulation of reins
(vii) Muscle output force adjustment tasks and sensory re-education training for motor ataxia
(viii) Low-frequency therapy on right wrist dorsiflexors (30 minutes daily)
(ix) Self-training focusing on stretching and reflex facilitation training for flexibility and adjustment of alignment of trunk and pinch movement training for extension and flexion of the right finger joints

Course

Regarding the patient's rein movements, motor ataxia was evident during reaching movements, and smooth opening and closing of the hand finger and total gripping of the reins were impossible because there was joint contracture in the ring finger. During rein manipulation, the trunk and scapula were unstable, the neck and trunk were being extended, and there was a risk of falling backward. We, therefore, provided rehabilitation aimed at (i) reducing joint contracture and motor ataxia and smoothly holding the reins, (ii) improving gripping and holding of the reins by improving sensory and grip function, and (iii) improving stability of the trunk and scapula.

As a result, on Day 8, contracture of the ring finger was reduced and ROM improved, and the patient was able to hold reins smoothly. At this time, the patient herself also said that it was easier to open her fingers. On Day 10, improvement of the rein gripping sensation in the hand finger area was confirmed. At discharge, stability of the trunk and scapula during rein manipulation had improved, and manipulation with the upper limb peripheral part was possible. Also, knot tying with both hands, the movement of sitting up from the paralyzed side, and gripping a plastic bottle with the right hand were also possible, and, as shown in Table 7.3, marked improvement was observed especially in WMFT. The patient herself also fully understood the need for the rehabilitation program and self-exercise and worked hard throughout.

Discussion

The patient presented with moderate right upper limb hemiparesis and, in everyday life, used the right upper limb as an assistive hand, but there were also many ADL in which she could not use the right upper limb due to abnormal alignment of the trunk and scapula, right ring finger contraction, and sensory impairment. When we carried out NEURO-15 the first time to treat such conditions, improvement such as the attainment of eating movements with a chopstick-type self-help device and nail-cutting movements in addition to improvement of the upper limb motor function were possible. Following NEURO-15 for the second time, gripping a plastic bottle with the right hand, knot-tying with both hands, and rein gripping movements, which were the target movements, became possible due to further improvement in upper limb motor function and sensory function. We believe that, in this patient, NEURO-15 for the first time resulted in improvement in the disuse of physical functions and triggered a change in behavior, i.e., "using the paretic upper limb in daily life," while NEURO-15 for the second time brought about improvement in physical functions in a true sense, and the quality and frequency of use of the paretic upper limb and the extent of use increased.

The change in the cerebral cortical activity as a result of NEURO-15 lasts for several months after treatment and appears to be extended further through the continuation of rehabilitation. We believe that because we continued rehabilitation on a regular basis following discharge for the first time, the change in the cortical activity was maintained. We also believe that NEURO-15 for the second time resulted in increased effectiveness, bringing about further improvement in motor function. However, we believe that the effectiveness of NEURO-15 could not be fully demonstrated due to the presence of organic changes such as muscle atrophy, joint contracture, and joint deformity. It is, therefore, important to continue regular exercise (rehabilitation) to prevent and improve restriction of ROM and muscle atrophy. In the future, we intend to explain the need for regular self-exercise and rehabilitation after discharge as part of our discharge guidance. This patient has a history of depression, but there was no sign of any recurrence as a result of rTMS treatment.

It was judged, therefore, that it is safe to deliver rTMS treatment provided there are no symptoms of depression at the start of therapy.

Patient Impressions

> I am now able to extend my fingers and hand fairly well and so I have started using them a bit more in everyday life. I think I am also now able to grip reins. When I go home, I want to try it out. I am now able to wash my hands with both hands and can also tie knots. I would like to receive treatment again next year.

Conclusion

We treated this patient, who had already undergone NEURO-15, with NEURO-15 again, taking into consideration joint contracture of the ring finger, motor ataxia, and sensory impairment. As a result, hand finger opening and upper limb motor function showed improvement both subjectively and objectively compared with the first time, and the target movements also became possible. This suggests that carrying out NEURO-15 multiple times may be a useful therapeutic intervention for firmly establishing the change in the cerebral cortical activity and increasing improvement of motor function.

Case 4

A 56-year-old male patient for whom NEURO-15 not only improved motor function but also increased life motivation.

Medical History and Background

In September 2011 (at the age of 55), the right-handed patient developed cerebral infarction (due to right middle cerebral artery occlusion), with speech difficulties and weakness of the left side of the body when he got up. After being given preservative acute phase treatment at the neurosurgery department of a nearby general hospital, he was hospitalized in a convalescent rehabilitation hospital for approximately 2 months and given rehabilitation for left hemiparesis. However, since noticeable paresis of the left upper limb and hand finger remained, in February

2012, he was hospitalized in our hospital for intensive rehabilitation. The patient had no medical history. He used to belong to a soccer club and became an instructor while continuing to play actively and taught children soccer. He later assumed an administrative position and did desk work, but, after onset, he resigned from his post as elementary school principal and took leave. However, he planned to return to work the month after discharge from this hospital, and his reassignment to the education affairs department had been decided. He strongly wished for recovery and also showed signs of a loss of life motivation. He lives with his wife.

Pretreatment Physical Findings

[General physical findings] Height 181 cm, weight 73 kg.

[Consciousness] Clear

[Higher brain function] Mild generalized attention disorder and executive dysfunction are evident. Trail Making Test (TMT)-A score was 77 seconds, and TMT-B was stopped due to signs of altering attention during the test. During evaluation, his expression was stern, with downcast eyes, and he seemed slightly in a daze.

[Motor system] Marked hemiparesis accompanied by increased muscle tone is evident in the left upper limb and left hand finger. Upper limb BRS is equal to stage V, but compensatory movements are noticeable, and difficulties with coordinated movements were seen. Hand finger BRS is equal to stage IV, full extension is difficult, and adduction of the thumb during pinching movements was observed.

[Sensory system] No obvious decline

[Standing and walking] The patient is fully capable of walking independently both indoors and outdoors. There was no particular sign of increased muscle tone, and lower limb BRS was equal to stage V. However, the left lower limb provides less support, left ankle dorsiflexion is insufficient, and reduced clearance is observed.

[ADL] A reduction in shoulder girdle support and stability was observed, compensatory movements were noticeable, and, since putting arms through sleeves in confined spaces was difficult, assistance with upper-body dressing movements and bathing was required. However, the patient performed other movements independently.

Evaluation Results

The results of each evaluation performed between the time of admission and 6 months after discharge were as shown in Table 7.4.

Table 7.4 Evaluation results (Case 4)

Evaluation method/items		At admission	At discharge	4 wks after discharge	4 weeks after discharge
BRS	Left upper limb	V	V	V	V
	Left hand finger	IV	V	V	V
Ueda's 12-grade motor function test for hemiplegia	Left upper limb	10	11	10	10
	Left hand finger	7	10	10	10
MAS	Wrist flexor muscles	1	1	1	1
	Finger flexor muscles	1	1	1	8
FMA (upper limb)	Overall score	48	57	54	54
WMFT	15 tasks perf. time (seconds)	655.08	74.42	294.16	188.07
10 second test (times)	Grip and release	0	7	8	8
Grip strength (kg)		8.8	10.5	11.6	7

Pretreatment Image Findings

A low-density area in the right putamen to corona radiata was observed on the head plain CT.

Patient's Needs, Treatment Goal, and Treatment Plan

The patient strongly wished for recovery of upper limb hemiparesis, but his needs in real life were unclear and vague. Therefore, upon consultation with the patient himself, we set the treatment goal of "independence in upper-body dressing movements," for which he required assistance, and "putting gloves on smoothly," which required time when going out. Based on this, we adopted the hospital treatment plan of providing OT focusing on stretching and facilitation, while delivering low-frequency rTMS every day for 15 days.

Content of Rehabilitation Program

(i) Low-frequency (1 Hz) rTMS to the hand finger area of the primary motor cortex in the left (nonlesional) hemisphere (20 minutes twice daily)

(ii) Stretching aimed at increasing the extensibility and flexibility of the shoulder joint, elbow joint, wrist, and finger joint flexor muscles with special focus on the pectoralis major muscle, biceps brachii, flexor carpi radialis muscle, flexor carpi ulnaris muscle, flexor digitorum superficialis muscle, and flexor digitorum profundus muscle

(iii) Facilitation of upper limb and placing in recumbent position aimed at increasing stability of shoulder joint and elbow joint

(iv) Space holding movement training of upper limb: incorporating stretching as required, aimed at increasing shoulder girdle support and left upper limb endurance

(v) Wrist dorsiflexion movement training: with the addition of low-frequency therapy for 15 minutes each time, performed aiming at increasing the strength of the dorsiflexors. Having the patient perform dorsiflexion movements voluntary to coincide with the low-frequency contraction rhythm

(vi) Pronation/supination movement training: ring exercise, incorporating visual feedback

(vii) Pinch movements and object gripping training: peg, marble, and coin pinching movement training

(viii) Guidance on self-exercise, focusing on stretching upper limb proximal muscles and distal muscles, dexterity and isolated movements

Course

Motivation for rehabilitation of the upper limb and hand finger was high, and, from the day following admission, we provided rehabilitation to improve shoulder girdle support, stability, and endurance and rehabilitation focusing on the wrist and dexterity training including dorsiflexion movements and object gripping. As a result, from approximately Day 4 in hospital, slight hand finger extension with wrist dorsiflexion began to be observed, and the patient himself also started saying things like "It feels like it will move" and "my shoulder is lighter." At discharge, comments such as "I am now able to put my jacket on by myself," "I am now able to open my hand and grasp things," "It is easier to put gloves on," and "I can now put my socks on with both hands" were evident, and we were able to achieve the treatment goal. As shown in Table 7.4, marked improvement especially for the FMA hand finger item was observed. The patient himself also fully understood the need to carry out the rehabilitation program and self-exercise and worked hard throughout.

Discussion

This patient underwent rehabilitation focusing on PT and OT at a nearby hospital for 4 months after onset, but, since marked paresis of the left upper limb and right hand finger remained, he wanted proactive treatment for this, and this led to treatment with rTMS at our hospital.

The needs of this patient were “to get dressed independently” and “to put gloves on smoothly.” Lower body dressing movements were independent, but upper body dressing required assistance, as forced movements accompanied by compensation were obvious due to a reduction in shoulder girdle support, stability, and endurance. For this patient, whose reinstatement to the education affairs department from the month following discharge had been decided, independence in ADL was considered essential.

In view of this, we provided rehabilitation for attainment of the target movements. We were able to reduce compensatory movements and strengthen the proximal part by carrying out training to increase the support of the shoulder girdle portion, and upper-body dressing movements became possible and the patient became independent. Regarding the hand finger, since marked adduction of the thumb was evident during pinching movements, we corrected this to abduction of the thumb by incorporating visual feedback and positive feedback leading to self-exercise and doing exercises such as marble and coin pinching. Moreover, the patient was very motivated about the rehabilitation and demonstrated an attitude of actively working on each training task and self-exercise. It was observed that this kind of positivity also led to improvement in hand finger movements.

Patient Impressions

> Initially, I was concerned about the nature of rTMS treatment, but when the therapy started, these concerns also disappeared. Ultimately I could be treated without pain or discomfort.
>
> As the days go by, the function of my hand improves and I realize that I now feel I can use my hand in daily life. I learned that the good cycle where I use by my hand because I feel I can and its function improves because I use it is important. I am once again determined to ‘get back a left hand that works’ so I get back to my old self. I will work hard at rehabilitation to achieve this.

Conclusion

This patient strongly wished for recovery from upper limb hemiparesis but demonstrated a decrease in life motivation. On this occasion, the patient experienced a functional recovery which led to an improvement in ADL, and life motivation improved further as a result of carrying out NEURO-15. Functional improvement also led to the confidence to return to work.

Case 5

A 57-year-old male patient with right upper limb hemiparesis accompanied by limb ataxia whose handwriting ability improved as a result of NEURO-15.

Medical History and Background

In August 2009 (at the age of 55), the left-handed patient developed intracerebral hemorrhage (left thalamus), and right hemiparesis accompanied by ataxia, and aphasia occurred. After receiving conservative treatment at a nearby acute phase hospital, he was admitted to a convalescent rehabilitation ward. He underwent rehabilitation in hospital for approximately 3 months, and, once he became independent in walking and ADL, he was discharged and allowed to return home. He later received rehabilitation at this hospital on an outpatient basis approximately once monthly but was hospitalized in our hospital for the purpose of NEURO-15 aimed at further improving upper limb motor function. The patient had a history of hypertension and hyperlipidemia and was taking medication including antihypertensive and lipid-lowering agents. He lived with his wife, worked in company management, and remained in management after onset. His job required a high degree of dexterity with both hands, but he was doing his job to the extent he could using his hand on the nonparalyzed side.

Pretreatment Physical Findings

[General physical findings] Height 165 cm. Weight 62 kg. He was left-handed but had been eating and writing with his right hand before onset.

[Consciousness] Clear

[Higher brain function] No abnormality. MMSE score was 30/30.

[Cranial nervous system] No abnormality

[Motor system] Right hemiparesis (BRS equal to stage VI for upper limb, stage VI for hand finger) and thalamic motor ataxia were observed. Isolated movements of both the upper limb and hand were possible but were slow and clumsy. Support of the upper limb proximal portion was low, and there was a tendency for increased shoulder joint adduction and tension of the adductor muscles. High tension of the pectoralis major muscle, biceps bracchi, trapezius muscle, and latissimus dorsi muscle was observed. Reaching movements were forced and were movements accompanied by extension of the trunk to increase stability, and spatial control of the upper limb was difficult. When pinching small objects such as pins or beans, the muscle tone of the thumb and index finger increased, and coordinated pinching with the finger pads was insufficient. In the finger-to-nose test, moderate tremor was observed, and motor ataxia tended to increase as a result of fatigue.

In movements of both hands in ADL such as washing face, tying tie, and putting on socks, the patient sometimes used the paretic hand as an assistive hand. However, manipulation of tools with the paretic hand was difficult, and the patient had no experience of using chopsticks with the paretic hand. Gripping a pencil with the paretic hand was possible, but handwriting was performed in a forced posture, involving lateral bending of the trunk to the nonparalyzed side. Distortion was evident in both straight and curved lines, and writing characters of the same size was also difficult (Fig. 7.1). MAS was 0 for shoulder, elbow, wrist, and finger joint flexor muscles. Deep tendon reflexes were (−) for upper limb and (−) for lower limb.

[Sensory system] Surface sensation was moderately dull in both the upper limb and hand finger. There was no clear decline in deep sensation, and the patient did not complain of numbness.

[Standing and walking] The patient was walking stably and independently both indoors and outdoors.

[ADL] The patient performed ADL, including taking a bath, independently. He took meals using chopsticks with the nonparetic upper limb and resting the paretic upper limb on the table. He could go out alone without any problem.

Evaluation Results

The results of each evaluation performed at admission and at discharge were as shown in Table 7.5.

Pretreatment Image Findings

A low-density area suggestive of old infarction lesion from the left thalamus/posterior limb of internal capsule to the left corona radiate is evident in head CT. Low-density areas were also observed in the white matter of bilateral frontal lobes, brain stem, and cerebellar vermis.

Table 7.5 Evaluation results (Case 5)

Evaluation method/items		At admission	At discharge
BRS	Right upper limb	VI	VI
	Right hand finger	VI	VI
FMA (upper limb)	Overall score	60	61
	Item A	34	34
	Item B	10	10
	Item C	14	14
	Item D	2	3
WMFT	15 tasks perf. time (seconds)	39.2	35.9
STEF		32	48
ICARS[a]		19	17

[a]ICARS (international cooperative ataxia rating scale)

Patient's Needs, Treatment Goal, and Treatment Plan

The patient's needs included "wanting to use right hand without tremor, wanting to eat something with chopsticks using right hand and wanting to write some letters with right hand." We, therefore, set "being able to eat all three daily meals using a chopstick-style self-help device in the right hand and being able to write more neatly" as treatment goals for him. Based on this, we adopted the hospital treatment plan of providing rehabilitation focusing on improving trunk and upper limb proximal portion support and improving upper limb and hand finger function, while delivering low-frequency rTMS to the nonlesional hemisphere on a daily basis.

Content of Rehabilitation Program

(i) Application of low-frequency rTMS (1 Hz) to the hand finger area of the primary motor cortex in the right (nonlesional) hemisphere (20 minutes twice daily every day).

(ii) Training to improve support of trunk and muscles surrounding the shoulder girdle: induction of movement of shoulder girdle accompanied by muscle activity of the abdomen aimed at improving isolated movements of the spine and shoulder girdle. Wrapping band around trunk to stabilize trunk and area surrounding shoulder girdle from the outside and to increase the activity of the upper limb.

(iii) Training to improve support of upper limb proximal portion: Gradual progression from holding therapy ball or rod on desk to holding upper limb in space, aiming for contraction of deltoid muscle, triceps brachii, and supraspinatus muscle. When shoulder joint adduction and tension of the adductor muscles tended to increase, we encouraged active movement, inducing movement manually. We also provided theraband exercises for the purpose of increasing activity of the rotator muscles.

(iv) Upper limb function training: repetitive training using objects, focusing on hand posture and reach, grasp, release. Intensive training of gross motor movement, gradually inducing trunk rotation and gradually changing the direction to sideward and backward and the distance.

(v) Dexterity training: handwriting training and repetitive training focusing on object manipulation tasks aimed at regaining coordinated muscle force output control of upper limb and hand finger. We used objects of varying sizes and materials including theraplast, building blocks, beanbags, and counters; gave feedback on the weightiness of the object; and sought adjustment of muscle force output.

(vi) Self-exercise guidance: provided immediately after intensive OT (60 minutes twice daily). Consisted in training to improve proximal portion support according to training described above followed by dexterity training.

We increased experience of perceptual exploratory activities from peripheral portion by focusing on activity of rolling and unrolling newspaper, handwriting training, and dexterity training using paretic hand. Practice using chopstick-style self-help device was implemented at actual mealtimes.

Course

From the day following admission, we provided rehabilitation focusing on training to improve support of the trunk and upper limb proximal portion and dexterity training. On Day 6, the patient began making comments like "I was not able to sense the weight and feel of objects before, but sensation around my thumb is clearer and my hand is now more stable." The patient also fully understood the need for the rehabilitation program and self-exercise and worked hard throughout. At discharge, the patient was able to eat all three daily meals using a chopstick-style self-help device in his paretic hand, and also in his handwriting, both straight lines and curved lines were less distorted (Fig. 7.14). The patient himself said that "My hand is easier to use now than when I was admitted," and he was motivated to train by himself after his discharge. As shown in Table 7.5, ICARS improved from a score of 19 to 17, and STER improved from a score of 32 to 48.

Discussion

Motor ataxia due to thalamic lesion is called thalamic ataxia and is characterized by the occurrence of motor ataxia on the opposite side of the thalamic lesion. Thalamic ataxia has reportedly been found in approximately 25 % of stroke patients with thalamic lesion, but these are often considered divided into three types: those accompanied by motor paralysis (ataxic hemiparesis), by sensory disturbance, and by both. In most patients presenting thalamic ataxia, disturbance of the ventrolateral thalamic nucleus is observed, and it is understood that thalamic ataxia occurs because the dentatorubrothalamic tract, which is formed by efferent fibers from the cerebellum, is damaged.

Since this patient presented ataxia accompanied by motor paralysis and sensory disturbance (hypesthetic ataxichemiparesis) due to thalamic lesion, he could not use the paretic upper limb and hand finger as a functional hand, though capable of isolated movements to some degree. He also had no choice but to go about his daily life without using his paretic hand, to prevent his trembling hand from being seen at work or when eating out.

When manipulating objects, this patient increased movements to compensate for reduced upper limb support, and coordination of agonist and antagonist muscles was difficult. He was, therefore, unlikely to be able to perceptually explore information from the peripheral portion, rendering proper regulation of muscle output force

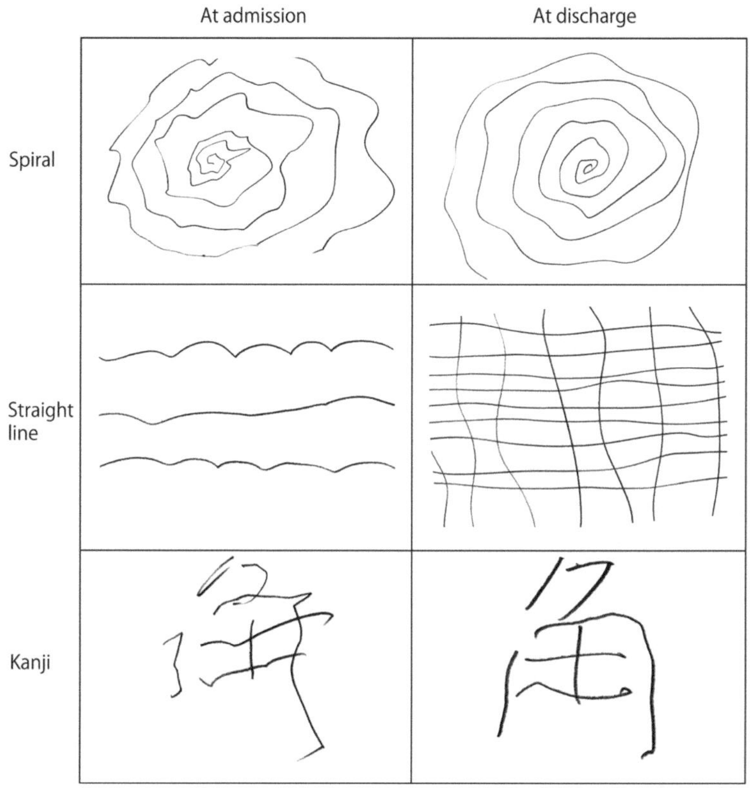

Fig. 7.14 Comparison of handwriting at admission and at discharge

and direction of movement and upper limb control difficult. We, therefore, thought that it was necessary to improve the support of the proximal portion of the upper limb and gradually increase selective use experience of the hand.

More specifically, we wrapped a band around the trunk to stabilize the unstable muscles surrounding the shoulder girdle from outside and then undertook object manipulation. We also incorporated a great deal of theraband exercise and object manipulation performed while checking the resistance and weightiness of the objects. Through these trainings, we expected to draw out selective and smoother movements of the hand based on the provision of feedback both visually and tactually. As a result, flexibility of the muscles and support of the upper limb were obtained, and coordinated movement of the upper limb and hand finger was better than before. We believe that in fact isolated movements were possible and we were, therefore, able to start object manipulation training using many tools, and muscle training from an early stage also has a positive impact on improvement of upper limb function.

It is noteworthy that, as a result of improvement of hypertonia in the forearm and hand finger during exercise, this patient commented that “sensation around the thumb was clearer" and "it was easier to use my hand." This is presumably because plastic changes accompanying the release from interhemispheric inhibition induced by rTMS facilitated coordinated movement of the upper limb and created a situation more easy than perceptual exploratory activities from the peripheral portion. Based on this, we believe that reduction of compensatory movement and encouragement of selective movements of the hand which are facilitated in intensive OT resulted in increased ability to perceive resistance from objects. This enabled control of muscle force output in the upper limb and hand finger according to the object and appears to have led to improvement in the manipulation efficiency of the hand finger. rTMS appears to be effective for the treatment of thalamic ataxia. However, further research into whether stimulation to the motor center of the hand or the cerebellum is more effective is expected in the future.

Patient Impressions

> I was able to concentrate entirely on my own body for two weeks and I have since been more motivated about self-exercise. I was able to confront this illness with a positive frame of mind. At home, I am eating meals using the chopstick-style self-help device introduced to me by the hospital.

Conclusion

We made use of this patient's comparative ability to perform isolated movements, and, from an early stage, we provided training to improve support of the upper limb proximal portion and dexterity training using objects, in combination with rTMS treatment. As a result, object manipulation speed, pinching movements, and ataxia when using tools improved. This suggested that NEURO-15 can be a useful therapeutic intervention for improving not only upper limb hemiparesis but also ataxia of the limb.

Case 6

A 49-year-old male patient whose phonological processing has improved as a result of rTMS on the right inferior frontal gyrus of frontal lobe.

Medical History and Background

In March 2009 (at the age of 49), the right-handed patient developed cerebral infarction (extensive infarction in the territory of the left middle cerebral artery), and aphasia and right hemiparesis occurred. He was taken to a university medical center in the Kanto suburbs, and after receiving acute phase medical care at this center, he underwent ST on an inpatient and outpatient basis at a convalescent rehabilitation hospital. In October 2009, he was examined at this hospital for the purpose of rTMS treatment. He then received ST on an outpatient basis roughly once weekly, and, in September 2010 (approximately 1.5 years after onset), he was hospitalized for 10 days of rTMS treatment. After completion of rTMS treatment, we continued to provide the patient with ST on an outpatient basis with the same frequency as before the therapy.

Before onset, the patient was a company employee (on leave during treatment) and lived with his wife and two children. He had no particular medical history.

Pretreatment Physical Findings

Although right hemiparesis was observed, in ADL, the patient walked independently outdoors using an ankle-foot orthosis and T-shaped cane. There was no clear evidence of dysarthria.

Pretreatment Speech and Higher Brain Function Findings

[Consciousness and general mental functions] While changes of facial expression and spontaneity appeared to be slightly poor, we judged that mental functions related to social contact had been more or less maintained. Regarding nonverbal intelligence, no marked decline was observed in tests, with a score of 34 in Raven's Colored Progressive Matrices test.

[Visual recognition] No abnormal findings

[Action] Slight buccofacial apraxia was observed (Only complex movements such as clicking of tongue were impossible).

[Speech] The results of this patient's standard language test of aphasia (SLTA) before rTMS treatment are shown in Fig. 7.15 (black dotted line). Although auditory comprehension was functional at least at a short-sentence level in everyday conversation, the tests showed a marked decline in comprehension of long sentences with complex structure (oral commands in SLTA). This was considered to be largely attributable to decline in linguistic short-term memory capacities (number counting: ± for three-digit numbers) and decline in syntactic comprehension.

There was marked decline in the quantity of speech, and, apart from standard questions and answers such as his name and "that's right" and "I don't know," almost no meaningful linguistic expression was observed. Likewise in tests, although the patient could name a number of familiar nouns (7/20 for "Naming" in the SLTA), explanation tasks at a sentence level ("Explain picture story," etc. in the

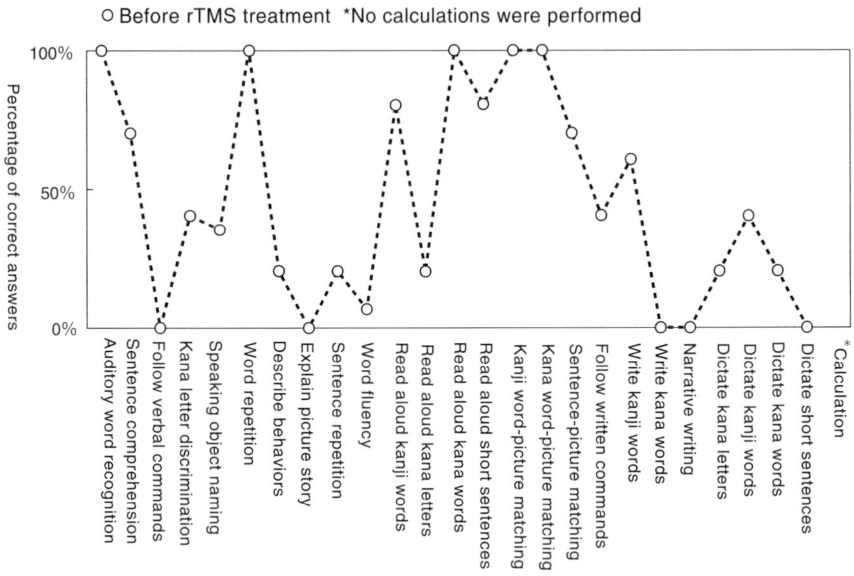

Fig. 7.15 SLTA results (1). Shows the patient's SLTA results before rTMS treatment

SLTA) ended in explanations such as "Like this, like this and then like this (while pointing to the picture)," and the decline in the quantity of information was severe.

As for the causal factors of speech disturbance, problems with multiple processes, including lexical selection, phonological processing, and syntax, were all considered to have a strong impact. In particular, the fact that situations in which the patient answered information about the mora (beats) of the target words, such as "three" or "quite a lot," even though he was unable to name them were seen frequently and the fact that initial sound hints for familiar nouns and verbs were extremely effective suggested clear difficulty in phonological recollection.

On the other hand, given that, in speech, almost no distortion of speech sounds could be heard and that there were almost no speech delays in sequential expressions such as standard questions and answers like those described above and counting from 1 to 10, we judged that anarthria is either not present or slight.

According to the tests, overall, comprehension of written language tended to be better than auditory comprehension. However, especially with regard to kana, although actual comprehension of easy words like those used in the SLTA was possible, reading aloud took time, and the patient demonstrated extreme difficulty reading aloud single kana letters and nonwords. Matching of vocal sounds and kana was also not easy.

Regarding writing, some simple single kanji words could be spontaneously written, and some could be dictated, but spontaneous writing of single kanji words was very difficult, and, also in dictation of vocal sound sequence presented by a tester, the patient was only able to write a very small part such as "HO-N," and there was a severe degree of disturbance.

Overall, the patient was considered to have aphasia characterized by moderate to severe disturbance of phonological fluency and disturbance linking vocal sounds and kana, severe syntactic disturbance (both in comprehension and expression), and moderate disturbance of lexical selection, and the total degree of aphasia was judged moderate to severe. While symptoms rendered clear classification difficult, broadly speaking, we perceived the patient's condition as falling between typical Broca's aphasia without elements of anarthria.

Pretreatment Image Findings

In head MRI images (TI-weighted images), an extensive low-intensity area from the middle frontal gyrus, inferior frontal gyrus, precentral gyrus, postcentral gyrus of left frontal lobe, supramarginal gyrus of parietal lobe, and superior temporal gyrus of temporal lobe to the deep white matter and lateral part of basal ganglia was observed, and, in functional MRI (fMRI) during language tasks, activation in the middle frontal gyrus and inferior frontal gyrus of left frontal lobe was confirmed (Fig. 7.16).

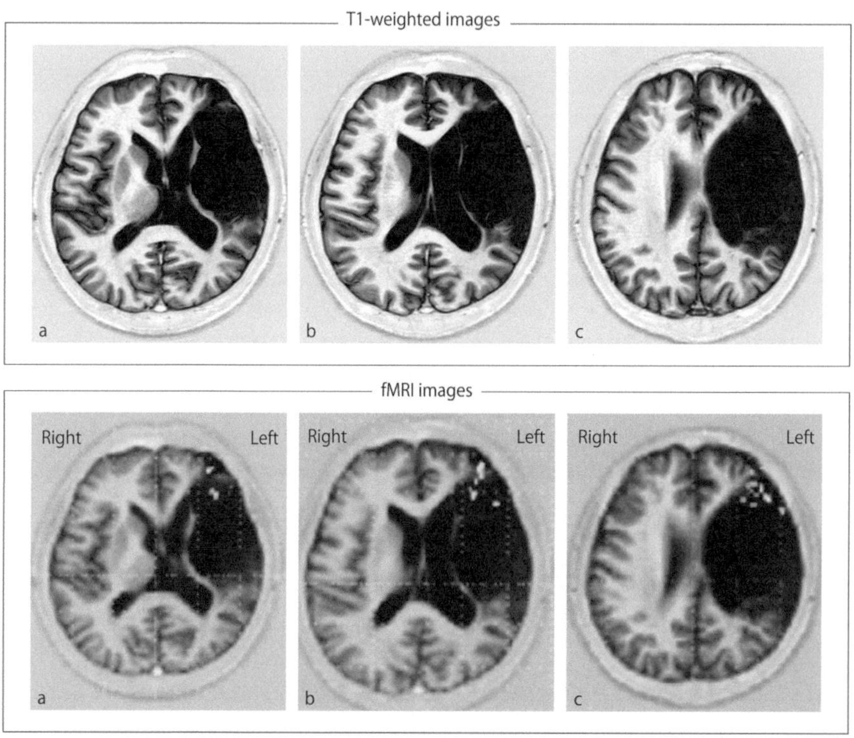

Fig. 7.16 Pretreatment image findings (Case 6)

Patient's Needs, Treatment Goal, and Treatment Plan

The need of this patient was to improve everyday communication skills as much as possible ahead of the fast-approaching time limit for his return to work. However, as things stood, expression at a single-word level was difficult, as stated in pretreatment speech findings.

In view of this, we set a long-term ST objective (in several years' time, including rTMS treatment) of "communicating short sentences that include a noun and a verb and have a concrete meaning" and a short-term objective (in several months' time) of "communicating information by expressing nouns or verbs that have concrete meaning at a single word level."

We adopted the treatment plan of "first aiming, as a top priority, for improvement in phonological recollection, which though severely disturbed is considered essential for expression at a single word level, and carrying out training with respect to the lexical selection process and syntax, as an extension of this."

Content of Rehabilitation Program

(i) Application of low-frequency (1 Hz) rTMS to the right inferior frontal gyrus (40 minutes per session for 10 days).

(ii) Provision of one-to-one ST for approximately 60–80 minutes each day (content during hospitalization for rTMS and during outpatient training before and after hospitalization is almost the same). Intervention focusing on phonological recollection and vocal sound and kana processing tasks in a broad sense in accordance with the aforementioned plan. Specific tasks included (1) vocal sound position in word identification and extraction tasks, (2) reversal of words with two to three moras that do not include special syllables, (3) construction of kana single words through selection from a group of kana characters containing dummies in response to pictures, (4) mora number recollection and naming with sound from end of or interior of word as a hint in response to pictures, and (5) reading aloud short sentences.

(iii) Distribution of printouts for self-exercise, with same content as for one-to-one ST (especially task of constructing kana single words through selection and copying from a group of characters).

Short-Term Evaluation Results

Table 7.6 shows this patient's speech function evaluation results directly before and after rTMS treatment. Before therapy is before the start of treatment on the first day after admission, and after therapy is the evaluation on the final day, directly after

Table 7.6 Evaluation results (Case 6)

Evaluation method/items			Before therapy	After therapy
SLTA-ST (assistive test)	Naming (no. of correct answers out of 40 words)[a]		12	10
	Explain picture story (Graded assessment: 6 is highest out of 6 grades)	1. Angler	2	2
		2. Chestnut tree	2	2
		3. Black cat and white cat	1	1
		4. Bird and whale	1	2
WAB	Repetition (score out of a total of 100)		40	44

[a]"Naming" in SLTA-ST is performed before and after treatment by splitting 80 words into two groups (40 words each) with no difference in the percentage of correct answers, with reference to the percentage of correct answers of 253 patients with aphasia and others at the time of test preparation shown in the manual

completion of the entire treatment schedule. In "Explain picture story" of the supplementary tests for standard language test of aphasia (SLTA-ST), although improvement in the graded evaluation was evident for one item only, overall, there was no substantial change.

Long-Term Evaluation Results

Figure 7.17 shows this patient's SLTA profile before and after rTMS treatment and approximately 1 year later. In this case, before therapy is directly before admission, and after therapy is 3 months after discharge. In the evaluation after therapy, the items that show clear improvement were the three items "Speaking Object naming," "Read aloud kana letters," and "Write kana words."

Course

As shown by the evaluation results, there was no significant change in symptoms during rTMS treatment in hospital or immediately after treatment, and the patient himself also sometimes stated (in the form of a Yes-No question) that "since my stroke onset, I feel that, whatever I do, my symptoms are, if anything, getting rapidly worse."

However, from approximately 2 to 3 months after therapy, the naming of high-frequency nouns, which was used in tasks, became easier, and the patient was increasingly able to name things immediately even without recalling the number of moras and hints. At the same time, situations in which the reading aloud and writing of kana, which was difficult before, gradually became possible began to be seen

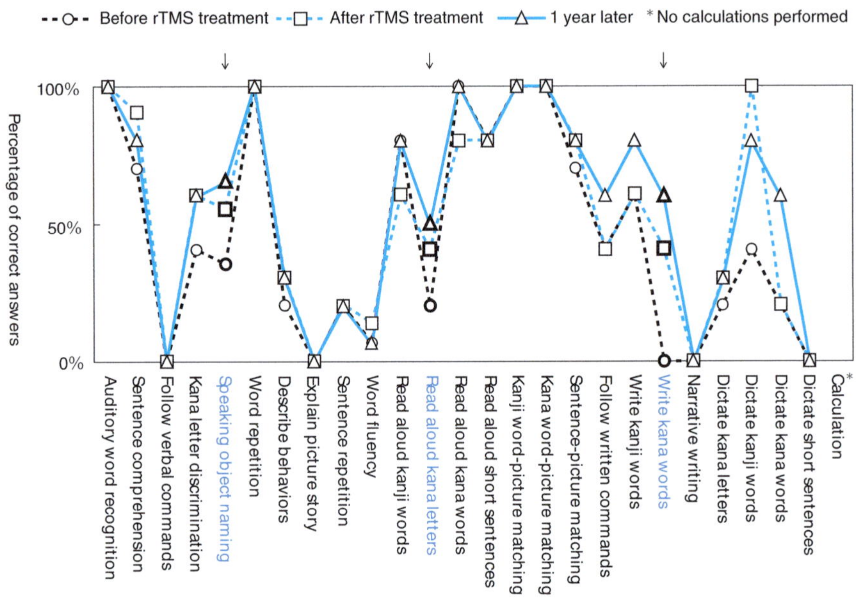

Fig. 7.17 SLTA results (2). Shows the patient's SLTA profile before and after rTMS treatment and approximately 1 year later

frequently. In the SLTA 3 months after therapy (Fig. 7.17) (blue dotted line), a clear change was observed, with the outcome for "Naming" improving from 7/20 words to 11/20 words and the patient smoothly writing 2 words in "Kana single word writing," which had been completely impossible before. Moreover, in "Naming," whereas the 7 words correctly answered before therapy were all grade 5 according to the scoring standard (correct answer from 4 seconds), in the SLTA after therapy, 10 out of the 11 correctly answered words were grade 6 (correct answer within 3 seconds), indicating a marked change in quality. However, on the other hand, difficulty naming low-frequency words remained the same as at the time of the test before therapy.

Later, also in everyday conversation, expression of meaningful single words was facilitated, and also in outpatient ST, the patient became able to progress to training in new areas such as tasks relating to the semantic lexical selection process and tasks relating to syntax. Figure 7.17 also shows SLTA scores after 1 year (blue solid line), and "Naming" and kana-related items which showed clear improvement after 3 months had almost all improved further after 1 year.

In terms of life, thanks to his company's generous support system, the patient gradually achieved a return to work from approximately 4 months after rTMS treatment. Initially, his duties consisted of non-language-type duties (e.g., delivering postal items to each department within the company) but later expanded to include duties such as numerical input into spreadsheet software using a computer.

Discussion

While there is a great deal of literature reporting improvement in naming as an effect of rTMS treatment in patients with aphasia, there is almost no literature that goes as far as mentioning the processes in which this improvement takes place in light of the cognitive-neuropsychological models for naming which we, as clinicians including speech therapists, use on a daily basis.

In this patient, the pattern of this improvement in naming was characterized not by the fact that the score for naming low-frequency words, whereby the word itself is difficult to identify, improved but by the fact that the patient became able to quickly and reliably name high-frequency words. Given that reading aloud and writing of kana improved at the same time, the marked improvement in language function gained during the 3 months or so after rTMS treatment can be considered to relate mostly to phonological recollection.

For this patient, since disturbance of phonological recollection and the need to improve this were already clear right from the outset, at the time of the initial evaluation, we provided training focusing on this prior to the initiation of rTMS treatment. As an underlying mechanism of improvement in this case, it is considered that the combined use of rTMS treatment and ST synergistically improved the outcome, as the target site of the rTMS determined based on the results of the fMRI and the effect of rTMS were perfectly consistent with the speech training plan.

Conclusion

For this patient, improvement in disturbance of phonological recollection and the related processes of naming and kana reading aloud and writing was observed over a comparatively long period as a result of the combined use of rTMS on the right inferior frontal gyrus of frontal lobe and ST. For this patient, we felt that rTMS treatment may have acted as a catalyst for long-span ST in the chronic phase.

Case 7

A 78-year-old male patient for whom bilateral rTMS and intensive swallowing rehabilitation were undertaken as a treatment for dysphagia after medullary infarction.

Medical History and Background

In April 2011 (at the age of 77), the right-handed patient presented with trunkal ataxia and dysphagia. He was diagnosed with medullary infarction and urgently admitted to a nearby general hospital. After undergoing conservative treatment, he was able to walk independently, but the dysphagia remained and he was, therefore, discharged home from hospital in a fasting state, having undergone gastrostomy. Although he subsequently underwent outpatient dysphagia rehabilitation at the same hospital, no improvement of swallowing functions was observed. Consequently, in March 2012, he visited our hospital's outpatient department and began to receive outpatient dysphagia rehabilitation once weekly, including stretching with a balloon. However, endoscopic evaluation of swallowing showed failure of initiation of the swallowing reflex and saliva aspiration, and oral intake remained difficult. Therefore, in June 2012, the patient was hospitalized for 7 days for the purpose of rTMS treatment for dysphagia. The patient had no particular medical history. He was taking antiplatelet agents. He lived with his wife.

Pretreatment Physical Findings

[Consciousness] Clear. No major abnormality with higher brain function.

[Swallowing function] Choking and wet hoarseness are observed as a result of the intake of thickened water.

[Motor system] There is no clear motor paralysis of the four limbs. The patient is stable standing and walking.

[Sensory system] There is thermal hypoalgesia of the right side of the face and left upper and lower limb.

[ADL] Independent

Evaluation Results

The results of each evaluation performed at admission and at discharge were as shown in Table 7.7.

Pretreatment Image Findings

A low-density area indicating an old infarction lesion in the right lateral medullary region was observed on a head plain CT. In addition, videofluorgraptic (VF) examination using barium jelly revealed failure of initiation of the swallowing reflex,

Table 7.7 Evaluation results (Case 7)

Evaluation method and evaluation items	At admission	At discharge
MASA[a]	149	161
P-A scale[b]	4	2
LEDT (seconds)[c]	3.22	1.2
SWAL-QOL (over-all)[d]	611	619
RSST[e]	1	2
FOIS[f]	1	2

[a]MASA (Mann assessment of swallowing ability)
[b]P-A scale (penetration-aspiration scale)
[c]LEDT (laryngeal elevation delay time)
[d]SWAL-QOL (the swallowing quality of life)
[e]RSST (repetitive saliva swallowing test)
[f]FOIS (functional oral intake scale)

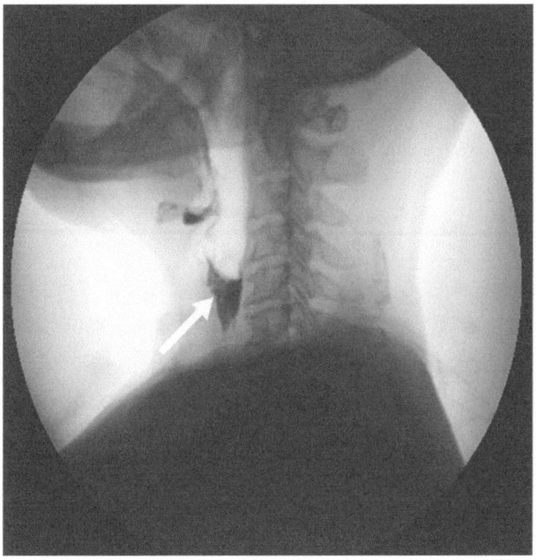

Fig. 7.18 Pretreatment image findings (Case 7) Pharyngeal residues of barium are observed in VF

obstruction of the esophageal orifice, pharyngeal residue, and saliva aspiration after swallowing (Fig. 7.18).

Patient Needs, Treatment Goal, and Treatment Plan

The need of this patient was “to become able to eat all three daily meals by mouth.” However, as things stood, dysphagia was severe, and, upon consultation with the patient himself, we, therefore, set the treatment goal as “intake of small amounts of semisolid food.” Based on this, we adopted the treatment plan of providing dysphagia rehabilitation focusing on indirect swallowing training in the pharyngeal stage, while delivering rTMS treatment on a daily basis.

Content of Rehabilitation Plan

(i) Application of rTMS (3 Hz) to the pharyngeal area of the bilateral primary motor cortex (10 minutes twice daily).
(ii) Head-raising training: lying in supine position with shoulder on floor and raising head only until toe is visible. "Raising continuously for one minute and then resting for one minute" three times through. If pulse is 120 beats per minute directly after raising, load is adjusted to prevent this.
(iii) Balloon stretching training: "Simple withdrawal technique" which involves swallowing 14 Fr Foley catheter and then inflating and withdrawing balloon is repeated five times per training session.
(iv) Exercising of tongue muscles focusing on dorsum of tongue raising training to increase pharyngeal pressure.
(v) Guidance to complete balloon stretching training for approximately 1 hour and 30 minutes twice daily as self-exercise.

Course

We began rTMS and dysphagia rehabilitation with a speech therapist from the day of admission. As a result, from approximately Day 4 in hospital, the swallowing reflex began to appear slightly easier, and the patient himself also started to say things like "I cough up less saliva." At the time of discharge, the daily amount of tissues necessary to wipe up coughed up phlegm had decreased, and also in the evaluation results shown in Table 7.7, marked improvement especially in the LEDT item was seen, and direct swallowing training using a small amount of jelly was possible. The patient himself also fully understood the need to carry out the rehabilitation program and the self-exercise and worked hard throughout.

Discussion

This patient presented with failure of initiation of the swallowing reflex and obstruction of the esophageal orifice, and aspiration of saliva was also often evident, and he was, therefore, a case in which safe oral intake was difficult. When we delivered rTMS and dysphagia rehabilitation, including balloon stretching, to treat these conditions, unfortunately, on this occasion, our intervention during his time in hospital alone was not enough to lead to the oral intake of all three daily meals. However, since clear improvement in swallowing initiation speed was achieved, this can be considered a step closer to safe oral intake.

While cricopharyngeal myotomy is sometimes considered to treat obstruction of the esophageal orifice as a result of medullary infarction, in cases where initiation of swallowing is difficult, the oral intake rate after surgery is low, and so surgery is often not indicated. Likewise in this patient, if balloon training proves unsuccessful, indication of surgery for improving function of swallowing will be considered, but then failure of initiation of swallowing will be a problem. Accordingly this time, when proposing the treatment program, we decided to prioritize improvement of failure of initiation of swallowing and subsequently to consider surgery to improve swallowing function.

That said, there is also the possibility that if we apply low-frequency rTMS to the cricopharyngeal muscle, the obstruction will be reduced, and swallowing function will be further recovered. In the future, we believe it is necessary to examine ways of selective rTMS, paying careful attention to individual cases.

Patient Impressions

As a result of receiving rTMS treatment, the swallowing reflex became easier to occur and the amount of phlegm decreased. In the future, I intend to consider surgery while continuing rehabilitation on an outpatient basis.

Conclusion

When treating this patient, we focused on failure of initiation of the swallowing reflex and provided dysphagia rehabilitation, consisting mainly of training in the pharyngeal phase, in combination with rTMS. As a result, speed of initiation of the swallowing reflex and aspiration of saliva showed improvement both subjectively and objectively. Therefore, combined approach to pharyngeal phase dysphagia rehabilitation and rTMS appeared to be a useful intervention in patients with dysphagia after medullary infarction.

Chapter 8
Future Challenges of rTMS Treatment

1 Combination Treatment of Botulinum Toxin Injection and rTMS Treatment (Naoki Yamada, Wataru Kakuda and Masahiro Abo)

A. What Is Botulinum Toxin Type A?

Clostridium botulinum is the generic name of the bacterium that produces botulinum toxin, and based on differences in the antigenicity of this toxin it is classified into seven types, namely, into type A to G. In 1977, an American ophthalmologist [1] succeeded in treating strabismus by using botulinum toxin type A (BoNT-A) as nonoperative treatment. As a result, BoNT-A began to be used in clinical practice for the treatment of various diseases such as "blepharospasm," "hemifacial spasm," "spasmodic torticollis," and "upper and lower limb spasticity."

From the end of the late 1990s, BoNT-A was widely used in the Western countries for the treatment of upper limb spasticity. In Japan, the use of BoNT-A was finally approved in October 2010 (through the expansion of the indications for its use, which since then also includes upper and lower limb spasticity). For the management of spasticity, it is important to perform BoNT-A therapy combined with rehabilitation. As of December 2012, Botulinum toxin type A products for the treatment of upper and lower limb spasticity that are covered by health insurance in Japan are limited to Botox® which is manufactured by GlaxoSmithKline. Therefore, the use of the signage BoNT-A in this chapter refers only to Botox®.

In vivo Botox® acts on cholinergic peripheral nerves and reduces muscle tonus by inhibiting the release of the neurotransmitter acetylcholine at neuromuscular junctions. Inhibition of the release of acetylcholine causes axonal sprouting in the vicinity of motor nerve endings at which neurotransmission is blocked through this toxin. Sprouting produces collateral axonal branches that repair endplates, thus leading to the formation of new endplates [2]. This nerve regeneration process

M. Abo, W. Kakuda, *Rehabilitation with rTMS*,
DOI 10.1007/978-3-319-20982-1_8

requires 3 to 4 months, which corresponds approximately with the clinical efficacy period of Botox®.

B. Actual Administration of BoNT-A for the Treatment of Upper Limb Spasticity

Upper limb spasticity is typically characterized by flexed postural patterns such as illustrated in the so-called Wernicke-Mann posture (Fig. 8.1) and manifest, e.g., as adduction or internal rotation of the shoulder joint and flexion of the elbow, wrist, and finger joints (the forearm can be pronated or supinated). Obviously, upper limb spasticity affects ADL and reduces QOL [3, 4].

BoNT-A therapy is used for a relatively wide range of indications, and one can try it out if it is expected that "with this therapy upper limb spasticity can be alleviated, and that this will bring relief from pain, or lead to an improvement of some sort of passive or active motions, that also will result in an improvement of ADL and QOL." In patients with severe hemiparesis "facilitating the extension of a passive upper limb joint for reducing the care burden" could also be a treatment goal that is

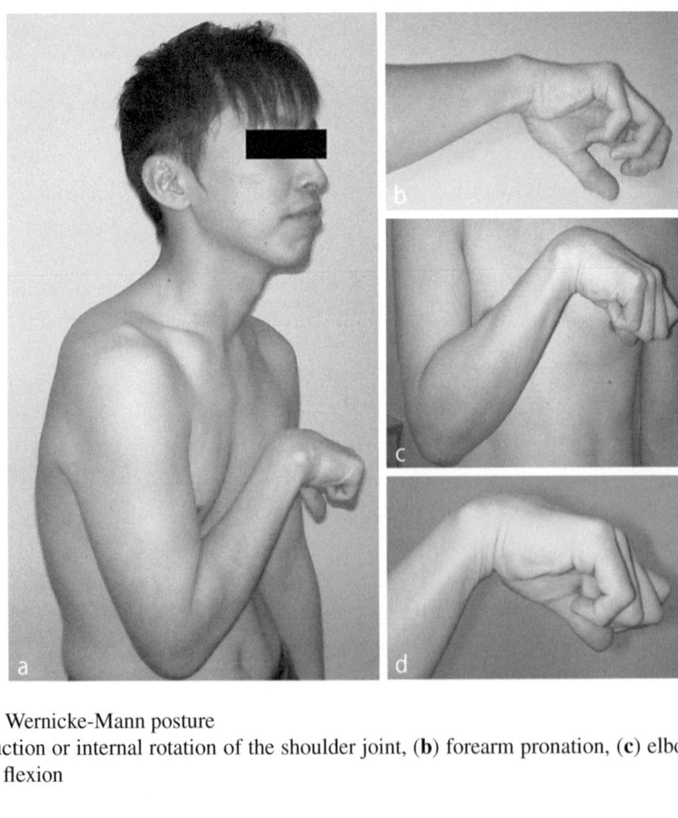

Fig. 8.1 Wernicke-Mann posture
(**a**) Adduction or internal rotation of the shoulder joint, (**b**) forearm pronation, (**c**) elbow flexion, (**d**) wrist flexion

worth to try out this therapy. Pronounced joint contracture and muscle atrophy are no indication for aggressive BoNT-A therapy, but in either case BoNT-A should be administered after having clarified "what treatment goal shall be achieved by its administration."

The muscles into which BoNT-A is injected are "muscles with increased tone that cause these abnormal postures." Therefore, depending on the individual condition of the patient, often four to six muscles are selected for treatment. In particular the following six muscles, namely, the "flexor carpi radialis muscle," "flexor carpi ulnaris muscle," "flexor digitorum profundus muscle," "flexor digitorum superficialis muscle," "flexor pollicis longus muscle," and "adductor pollicis muscle," play an important role in BoNT-A therapy and have also been investigated in studies on BoNT-A therapy that were conducted in Japan. However, in cases with pronounced adduction or internal rotation of the shoulder joint or elbow flexion, BoNT-A is also injected into the "pectoralis major muscle," "latissimus dorsi muscle," and "biceps brachii muscle."

The dose of BoNT-A is determined depending on the degree of spasticity and the volume of muscle into which it is injected. In the case of large muscles such as the pectoralis major muscle or biceps brachii muscle 50–100 units are appropriate, and in the case of other upper limb muscles up to 50 units are considered appropriate. However, at present in Japan, the administration of BoNT-A for the treatment of upper limb spasticity is only covered by health insurance up to a maximum dose of 240 units.

It is not necessary to search for the motor points of the muscles when injecting BoNT-A into muscles of the upper limb. It is likely that a muscle relaxing effect is achieved if the injection needle was inserted into the muscle belly and BoNT-A was unmistakably injected into the muscle. Normally after 2 to 7 days an antispasticity effect is observed, and although there are individual differences, this effect is sustained for approximately 3 to 4 months. It is possible to repeat administration 3 months or more after injecting BoNT-A; however, in this case the original degree of spasticity often returns if the injection of BoNT-A is not used in combination with rehabilitation. In case of upper limb spasticity it is possible to gradually regain the original softness of the muscles by combining treatment with BoNT-A with OT, and we have experienced that lower doses are required for repeated BoNT-A treatment.

As for adverse reactions, it is believed that the possibility of serious complications is very low if upper limb spasticity is being treated by use of BoNT-A, but sometimes an excess muscle relaxing effect is observed (in particular, if, e.g., high doses of BoNT-A were administered compared to the degree of spasticity).

For the main injection sites and methods used when injecting BoNT-A into muscles of the upper limb please refer to Table 8.1. Moreover, based on our experience we have summarized important points and precautions regarding BoNT-A therapy for the treatment of upper limb spasticity in Table 8.2. However, it is not rare that patients think that "after injection of BoNT-A upper limb hemiparesis will improve without fail and that there will be no need to perform rehabilitation," and therefore the goal of BoNT-A therapy and the necessity of concomitant rehabilitation should be sufficiently explained to the patient prior to administration.

Table 8.1 Injection sites and treatment methods used when injecting BoNT-A into major muscles of the upper limb

Name of muscle	Site of injection and method
Pectoralis major muscle	The arm is abducted at the shoulder joint, and the injection needle is inserted while grabbing the muscle together with the subcutaneous fat layer
Biceps brachii muscle	The forearm is supinated, and the injection needle is inserted into the muscle belly in the middle of the upper arm
Brachioradialis muscle	The forearm is pronated, and the injection needle is inserted into the middle point between the biceps brachii tendon and the lateral middle condyle of the humerus
Flexor carpi radialis muscle	The injection needle is inserted approximately 4–5 cm distal to the middle point between the biceps brachii tendon and the medial epicondyle of the humerus
Flexor carpi ulnaris muscle	The injection needle is inserted two fingerbreadths volar to ulnar at a height 1/3 proximal to the forearm
Flexor digitorum superficialis muscle	The forearm is supinated, and the injection needle is inserted through the flexor carpi radialis muscle at the palmar side of the forearm
Flexor digitorum profundus muscle	The elbow is flexed, the forearm is supinated, and the injection needle is inserted 3–4 fingerbreadths distal to the olecranon
Flexor pollicis longus muscle	The injection needle is inserted through the flexor carpi radialis muscle and the flexor digitorum superficialis muscle in the middle of the forearm
Adductor pollicis muscle	The injection needle is inserted into the first interdigit towards the base of first metacarpal bone

Table 8.2 Important points and precautions regarding BoNT-A therapy for the treatment of upper limb spasticity

1.	First the goal of BoNT-A injection (e.g. relief of pain, improvement of passive and active motions) should be clarified. Then this should also be explained to the patient (and the patient's family)
2.	The dose of BoNT-A is determined depending on e.g. the size of the muscle into which it is injected, and the degree of spasticity, however, there are individual differences regarding its efficacy
3.	The patient (and the patient's family) should be fully explained that it is desirable that also after BoNT-A injection rehabilitation (OT) is conducted
4.	The rehabilitation program following BoNT-A injection should be determined depending on the condition of upper limb spasticity of the individual patient
5.	Self-exercise of the upper limb is an important part of rehabilitation following BoNT-A injection
6.	When some sort of rehabilitation intervention for the treatment of upper limb hemiparesis is being performed, and it is judged that the implementation of this rehabilitation intervention is blocked by the spasticity, then BoNT-A should be injected prior to the intervention
7.	Even if the aim is only to improve passive motions, it is possible that in combination with rehabilitation the antispasticity effect of BoNT-A is amplified
8.	If following BoNT-A injection muscle weakness is observed, the patient should be provided sufficient explanation about his/her condition, and be followed up
9.	BoNT-A is an expensive drug, but BoNT-A therapy provides excellent "cost- effectiveness"

C. Use of BoNT-A in Combination with NEURO-15

As outlined in the book by Ward et al. [5], which was published in 2001, that "BoNT-A therapy should be performed in combination with rehabilitation," the concept that BoNT-A therapy should be performed in combination with rehabilitation has been advocated since a long time ago. Also in the International Consensus Statement by Sheehan et al. [6] in 2010 it is stated that "the treatment of upper limb spasticity should be addressed by a comprehensive approach the core of which is BoNT-A therapy," and moreover it is being recommended to combine BoNT-A therapy with rehabilitation.

In April 2008 we started to use low-frequency rTMS in combination with intensive OT at our department. This combination therapy, which we termed "NEURO," was devised by our group and is conducted over a period of 15 days. Since April 2009 we are actively using a 15-day combination treatment protocol termed "NEURO-15" for the treatment of poststroke upper limb hemiparesis. At the present stage, virtually in all patients in whom we tried this therapy, NEURO-15 could be safely completed, and regarding its therapeutic effect, significant improvement has been confirmed for FMA and the performance time of the 15 tasks of the WMFT. However, its therapeutic effect appears to be considerably affected by the degree of spasticity of the upper limb on the paralyzed side prior to treatment, and tends to wane the severer the degree of spasticity of the upper limb.

Therefore, we started a combination treatment in which upper limb spasticity is reduced by performing BoNT-A therapy prior to NEURO-15 [7]. Soon after the use of BoNT-A for the treatment of upper and lower limb spasticity was approved in October 2010, our group actively attempted to perform BoNT-A therapy in patients with spasticity of the upper and lower limb, and from the very beginning we considered it important to adhere to the concept that "BoNT-A therapy should be performed in combination with rehabilitation."

Below, we present "a patient successfully treated with BoNT-A therapy prior to the rehabilitation in order to enhance the efficacy of rehabilitation at the Department of Rehabilitation, Shimizu Hospital, The Kyosaikai Medical Foundation," based on the idea that the presence of spasticity might be an inhibitory factor of rehabilitation. Moreover, we present "motor function evaluation data of patients in whom BoNT-A therapy was performed in combination with NEURO-15" from the same department.

D. Actual Use of BoNT-A Combined with NEURO-15 (Presentation of a Patient in Whom This Treatment Was Remarkably Effective)

1) Medical History, Living Situation

This patient was a 49-year-old woman. In August 2008 she experienced intracerebral hemorrhage and was urgently admitted to a general hospital nearby with right hemiparesis (dominant hand) caused by left putamen hemorrhage. She received conservative medical treatment and was discharged in October of the same year. Until March 2009 she underwent rehabilitation including OT of the upper limb at the same hospital, but movement disorder of the right upper limb remained. Hereafter, she was provided day service and visiting rehabilitation. However, in September 2011 she was admitted to our department because her condition did not change, and she hoped that "her condition would improve at least a little." She lived together with her husband and two children, and before onset she had been a housewife. At present she mainly uses her left upper limb when carrying out household chores or cooking meals.

2) Physical Findings Before Treatment

Muscle tone of the whole upper limb was increased, and marked in particular during motion. She could neither extend nor relax her fingers, dorsiflexion of the wrist was only possible when extending her elbow, and was not seen when the elbow was flexed. Her wrist was in a contracted state.

Brunnstrom recovery stage (BRS) was stage IV for the upper limb and stage III for hand-finger, but no sensory disturbance was observed. Muscle tension was high in upper limb through the elbow to hand-finger, with MAS of 2–3. Flexion of all fingers and radial abduction of the thumb was slightly possible; however, when grasping objects all fingers were flexed, and the grasped object was clenched inside her hand, because she could not extend her fingers. FMA score for items in the upper limb section was 40 points, and performance time for 15 WMFT tasks was 1090 seconds.

3) The Needs and Treatment Goals of This Patient

The needs of this patient were to be able "to hold a rice bowl while eating," "to hold a cup when drinking liquids," "to eat with chopsticks," and "to write with her paralyzed hand." Therefore, treatment goals were set as follows: to reduce the muscle tone of the whole upper limb, to become able to extend her fingers (in particular the thumb and index finger), to gain pinching motions, to gain grasping movements necessary for holding a cup, and movements that are necessary for using chopsticks.

4) Course of Treatment

In Week 1 a rehabilitation was provided focusing on improving operability and stability of the central upper limb, and reduction of muscle tone of the distal upper limb. Increased muscle tone of the whole upper limb was treated by injecting BoNT-A on Day 3 of hospitalization (biceps brachii muscle: 50 units, flexor carpi radialis muscle: 25 units, flexor digitorum superficialis muscle: 25 units), and by performing mainly physical therapy and stretching exercises. From around the end of Week 1 a reduction in the muscle tone of the distal upper limb was observed, and she could also voluntarily relax her fingers.

In Week 2 mainly neuromuscular facilitation of the distal upper limb was performed. As for finger extension and dorsiflexion of the wrist, after spasticity of the finger, wrist, and palmar flexor muscle groups had been reduced, finger extension and dorsiflexion of the wrist were encouraged through neuromuscular facilitation. As for the fingers, in particular palmar abduction of the thumb and extension of the index finger were performed, and at the beginning of Week 2 extension of the thumb and index finger, and in the middle of Week 2 pinching motions became possible. At the end of the week the patient was able to eat with a pair of tweezers-shaped chopsticks. The goal to become able to grasp a cup was not achieved because the patient could not sufficiently extend her other fingers, but nevertheless the results of motor function evaluation had improved significantly.

At discharge, MAS was 0–1, FMA score for items in the upper limb section was 50 points, and performance time for 15 WMFT tasks was 558 seconds.

5) Discussion

When we started to treat this patient, 3 years had passed since the onset, and she had no rehabilitation for the previous 1 year. Therefore, a high degree of spasticity and mild contracture of the wrist was observed, and as a result of spasticity it was difficult for her to move the upper limb and fingers of the paralyzed side.

We believe that her motion could be facilitated because reduced spasticity resulted from our treatment focused on spasticity. It has been reported that reduced spasticity is the main factor that leads to the recovery of motor function. As a result of trying to achieve changes in motor function and to reduce spasticity, also in this patient reduced spasticity was observed prior to improvement in motor function. We believe that this treatment approach, in which the reduction effect that BoNT-A therapy and rTMS have on spasticity is combined with rehabilitation specifically designed for the treatment of spasticity, was remarkably effective in reducing spasticity and that this led to the recovery of motor function.

E. Actual Use of BoNT-A Combined with NEURO-15 (Presentation of Data)

A total of 67 poststroke patients who had a stroke more than 1 year before with upper limb hemiparesis (based on the eligibility criteria for NEURO-15) and obvious spasticity received injection of BoNT-A into the paralyzed upper limb (total dose was 100–240 units for, e.g., biceps brachii muscle, flexor carpi radialis and flexor carpi ulnaris muscle, flexor digitorum superficialis and flexor digitorum profundus muscle) within 3 days after initiation of treatment following hospitalization before NEURO-15.

At present in our department NEURO-15 consists of combination treatment with low-frequency rTMS for 40 minutes and intensive OT for 120 minutes over the 15-day hospitalization. We decided to apply in each low-frequency rTMS treatment session at 1-Hz for 40 minutes (total of 2400 pulses) to the hand-finger areas in the primary motor area of the unaffected hemisphere. One treatment session of intensive OT consisted of one-to-one training for 120 minutes and self-exercise for 120 minutes. The one-to-one training, which was conducted with an occupational therapist, was centered on shaping exercises and repetitive motion exercises. Motor function of the upper limb was evaluated by use of, e.g., FMA upper limb evaluation items, performance time for 15 WMFT tasks, and MAS.

As a result, no adverse reactions or adverse events related to BoNT-A injection or the implementation of NEURO-15 were observed in any of the patients. At the time when NEURO-15 was completed significant improvement was observed in FMA scores, performance time for 15 WMFT tasks, as well as MAS (elbow, wrist, and MCP flexor muscle group). The results of motor function evaluation before and after treatment are summarized in Table 8.3.

This shows that BoNT-A injection prior to NEURO-15 improved spasticity, which is an inhibitory factor of rehabilitation, and promoted the effectiveness of NEURO-15 (in particular of intensive OT), and that this eventually led to improved motor function. Therefore we believe that it is desirable that in the future, patients with upper limb hemiparesis who present with spasticity are treated with BoNT-A as a "pre-conditioning procedure" prior to NEURO-15, and rehabilitation interventions such as CIMT, and robot-assisted training for making it more easy for the patient to conduct these kinds of training.

We are actually examining whether BoNT-A therapy prior to NEURO-15 can improve the therapeutic effects for the motor function in patients with upper limb hemiparesis. We included 80 poststroke patients with upper limb hemiparesis whose BRS for hand-fingers were stage III to V and who received NEURO-15 through April 1, 2010, to January 20, 2013, at our affiliated and collaborative hospitals. All the subjects met the following criteria for inclusion:

(1) MAS of ≥1 for finger flexor muscles and/or wrist flexor muscles. (2) BRS for hand-fingers of 3–5 (ability, at least subjectively, to flex all fingers of the affected upper limb in full range of motion). (3) Age at intervention between 18 and 90 years. (4) Time between the onset of stroke and intervention of ≥12 months. (5) A

Table 8.3 Motor function evaluation results before and after combination treatment with BoNT-A and NEURO-15[a]

Evaluation method and outcome measures		Pre-treatment	Post-treatment	*P* value
MAS	Elbow flexor muscle group	1.55±0.82	1.06±0.70	<0.05
	Wrist flexor muscle group	1.51±0.89	0.79±0.74	<0.05
	MCP flexor muscle group	1.52±1.01	0.77±0.81	<0.05
FMA (upper limb)		36.6±12.2	42.5±12.5	<0.05
WMFT	15 Task performance time (seconds)	688.3±406.8	557.0±368.9	<0.05

[a]*N*=67, evaluation results are all expressed as mean±SD

single symptomatic stroke lesion confirmed with clinical examination and brain MRI (no bilateral stroke lesions). (6) No marked cognitive impairment. (7) No active physical or mental illness. (8) No recent history of seizure. (9) No documented epileptic discharge on pretreatment electroencephalography. (10) No pathological conditions known to be contraindications for rTMS in the guidelines suggested by Wassermann [8]. In addition, the following patients were excluded from the study: patients with contraindications for intramuscular injection on BoNT-A (e.g., preexisting neuromuscular diseases, bleeding disorders, allergy or hypersensitivity to the product), patients who had received BoNT-A injections previously, and patients with concomitant use of oral antispastic medication.

The examined subjects were divided into two groups: one included 42 patients who received BoNT-A beforehand (mean age: 62.9 ± 10.2 years old, mean time after stroke: 62.0 ± 51.7 months), and the other included 38 patients who did not receive BoNT-A beforehand (mean age: 57.2 ± 15.2 years old, mean time after stroke: 48.0 ± 29.8 months). During the 15-day hospitalization, each subject received 12 treatment sessions consisting of (1) low-frequency (1 Hz) transcranial magnetic stimulation for 40 minutes, (2) tailored occupational therapy for 120 minutes, and (3) self-exercise for 120 minutes. The group with prior administration received an intramuscular injection of BoNT-A before the first treatment session. MAS was used to evaluate the contracture level of the wrist and the finger flexor muscles, while FMA and WMFT were used to evaluate the upper limb function. Each patient was assessed before and after treatment. As a result, a statistically significant improvement in the upper limb function was observed at the time of discharge in both groups ($P<0.001$) from the time of hospitalization. The amount of change in MAS and FMA of finger flexor muscles in the group with prior administration of BoNT-A improved significantly compared to the group without prior administration ($P<0.05$).It was demonstrated that prior administration of BoNT-A can improve the therapeutic effect of NEURO by improving the upper limb spasticity [9].

2 Coadministration of Levodopa with rTMS (Naoki Yamada, Wataru Kakuda, and Masahiro Abo)

A. Mechanism of Action of Dopamine

Dopamine is a neurotransmitter that is present in the central nervous system and a precursor to adrenaline and noradrenaline. Neurons that release dopamine are called dopaminergic neurons, and among these there are dopaminergic cell groups called A8, A9, A10 that are considered to be involved in learning and the execution of movements. A8 cell group is located in the retrorubral field (RRF), A9 cell group in the substantia nigra pars compacta (SNc), and the dopaminergic A10 cell group in the ventral tegmetal area (VTA). The VTA forms a part of two dopaminergic pathways through which the nucleus accumbens is connected with the mesolimbic system, and the frontal lobe is connected with the mesocortical system.

The nigrostriatum, which is related to Parkinson's disease, was previously believed to be directly involved in motor control; however, then it was found that motor control is regulated via, e.g., the globus pallidus and substantia nigra pars reticulate [10, 11]. When the dopamine needs of the striatum are depleted due to the degeneration or loss of dopaminergic cells in the substantia nigra pars compacta, then this results in movement disorders that are mainly characterized by akinesis, rigidity, and tremor. When the excitatory input to cells of the direct pathway that arises from the striatum through the D1 receptor is reduced due to dopamine depletion, then these activities decrease, and neural activity of the internal segment of the globus pallidus is enhanced. In addition, when the inhibitory input to cells of the indirect pathway that arises from the striatum through the D2 receptor is reduced, then these activities decrease, and as a result neural activity of the external segment of the globus pallidus is reduced, and neural activity of the subthalamic nucleus and internal segment of the globus pallidus is enhanced. Through these mechanisms, neural activity of the internal segment of the globus pallidus and substantia nigra pars reticulate is enhanced, and as a result the activity of the thalamus and cerebral cortex is suppressed. Moreover, it has been found that the effects of dopamine on the nigrostriatal pathway are also related to the brain's reward system. It is believed that dopamine plays a role in learning to predict which rewards one can expect depending on one's actions.

A reduction in dopamine levels does not only cause motor function adjustment disorders but also greatly affects mental activity and learning function. Depending on the areas that were affected by the stroke these neural pathways can be directly or indirectly impaired, and cause symptoms similar to Parkinson's disease. Therefore, it is important to determine which site was impaired, and to carry out rehabilitation and promote dopamine secretion while taking consideration of emotional functions of the patient such as pleasure and discomfort and expected rewards. However, since the effects of rehabilitation are limited, it is important also to consider a drug therapy that facilitates dopamine secretion.

B. Oral Levodopa + NEURO-15

In 2001, in a double-blind RCT that involved 53 first-ever stroke patients, after daily low-dose levodopa (100 mg) for 3 weeks followed by rehabilitation, motor function was found to have been significantly improved compared to the placebo group [12].

Since orally administered dopamine cannot cross the blood–brain barrier, levodopa was used as a prodrug of dopamine (precursor). Levodopa crosses the blood–brain barrier by making use of the L-amino acid transport mechanism and is decarboxylated in neurons of the central nervous system to form dopamine. However, since after long-term levodopa therapy the effect of levodopa becomes shorter, a phenomenon that is called "wearing off," treatment is generally initiated with small doses of levodopa.

As described above, there are dopaminergic neurons that are profoundly involved in learning and the execution of movements, namely, cell groups A8, A9, and A10.

Through the oral intake of levodopa, the dopamine secretion of these neurons can be supplemented. When dopamine secretion is enhanced, overactive basal ganglia are suppressed, and this in turn suppresses excessive muscle tone and triggers smooth movements. Moreover, since dopaminergic neurons also influence functions of the frontal association area and limbic cortex, they also affect the setting in of motions, and psychophysiological and learning functions. Thus, through the performance of appropriate exercises, and by acting on the limbic system, which is that part of the brain that controls our emotions, autonomic dopamine secretion is promoted, and neural circuits that are involved in motor learning are reinforced.

Focusing on these effects of levodopa, we examined the safety and efficacy of oral intake of levodopa combined with rTMS treatment. In a study five poststroke patients with hemiparesis started oral administration of low-dose levodopa (100 mg) 1 week prior to 2-week hospitalization for NEURO-15 treatment and continued the medication through hospitalization to 4 weeks after discharge. This study was completed without observing any side effects, and a significant improvement in motor function was seen. After 4 weeks when evaluating motor function again this improvement was still sustained or an even greater improvement was observed [13]. We expect that in the future not only levodopa but also other drugs that are more effective and safely increase brain activity will be used in combination with rTMS.

3 Clinical Introduction of Other Stimulation Modalities

Classification of TMS

1) What Are Conventional and Patterned rTMS?

At present the application of rTMS is based on various theories, and depending on the stimulation method rTMS is roughly classified into two types as shown in Fig. 8.2.

Conventional regular rTMS is called "conventional rTMS," and irregular rTMS is called "patterned rTMS." Conventional rTMS stimulation is a method in which stimulation is repeated at regular intervals. Stimulation at a frequency of 1 Hz or less is defined as low-frequency rTMS, and 5 Hz and more is defined as high-frequency rTMS. As shown in Fig. 8.3, patterned rTMS includes TBS in which bursts of three pulses are repeated at high frequency (50 Hz), and quadri-pulse stimulation (QPS) [14]. It has been reported that QPS, in which bursts of four pulses are repeated, or changes in the stimulation interval, result in both facilitatory and inhibitory effects that are consistent with the synaptic plasticity response defined in the Bienenstock-Cooper-Munro (BCM) theory [15].

Low-frequency rTMS of conventional rTMS, cTBS of patterned rTMS, and QPS using long stimulus intervals (e.g. 50 ms) result in a prolonged inhibitory effect on output from the corticospinal pathway. On the contrary, high-frequency rTMS using conventional rTMS, iTBS of patterned rTMS (described below), and QPS at short stimulus intervals (e.g. 5 ms) result in a prolonged enhancing effect.

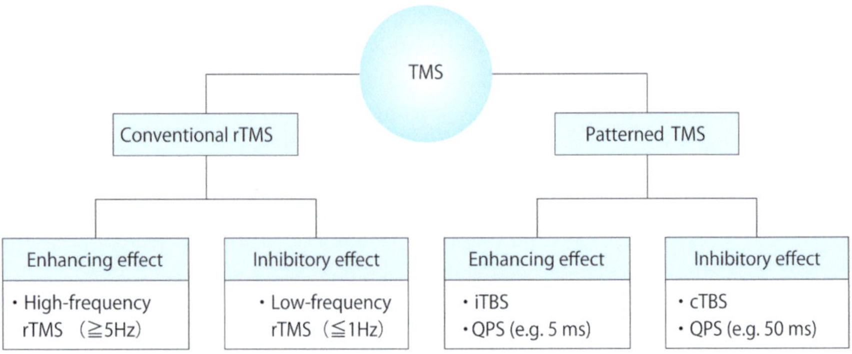

Fig. 8.2 Classification of TMS

2) What Is TBS?

Among various kinds of patterned rTMS, here we describe TBS, the clinical application of which is expected to further increase in the future. Huang et al. [16] reported that TBS can change the excitability of the human cerebral cortex within a short period of time, and in recent years, TBS which previously was only used in animal studies is increasingly also applied in humans, and research on the elucidation of its mechanism of action has advanced. The stimulation intensity used for TBS is only weak, namely, 80 % of the motor threshold of voluntary contraction. TBS consists of 3-pulse TMS trains at 50 Hz (TMS consisting of three pulses at intervals of 20 ms) that are repeated at regular intervals, in total 300–600 pulses. TBS stimulation methods include continuous TBS (cTBS), intermittent TBS (iTBS), and intermediate TBS (imTBS) (Fig. 8.3) [14].

Huang et al. reported that when using this method a short stimulation duration of only 40 seconds (cTBS) was sufficient to reduce the excitability of the cerebral cortex for approximately 60 minutes. In this report it is pointed out that conversely at the same intensity and same number of 600 pulses it is possible to enhance the excitability of the primary motor area when slightly changing these stimulation conditions. More specifically, the excitability of the cerebral cortex was enhanced when 3-pulse TMS at 50 Hz is repeated as 2-second train at frequency of 5 Hz every 10 seconds (total of 600 pulses). Reportedly with this method the excitability of the human cerebral cortex could be enhanced or reduced after only extremely short stimulation duration of 20–190 seconds, and the clinical application of this rTMS stimulation method is believed to hold promise for the future.

We then also conducted a pilot study which examined how TBS in combination with the intensive occupational therapy can improve the motor function in post-stroke patients with upper limb hemiparesis. We included 25 stroke patients in the chronic phase with upper limb hemiparesis (mean age: 62.2 ± 12.6 years old, mean time after stroke: 71.8 ± 63.6 months) who received inpatient treatment at Shimizu Hospital, one of our affiliated hospitals, for 15 days during the period from February 2 to December 21, 2013. Their BRS for upper limb and hand-fingers were III or more, and they had not received botulism in combination.

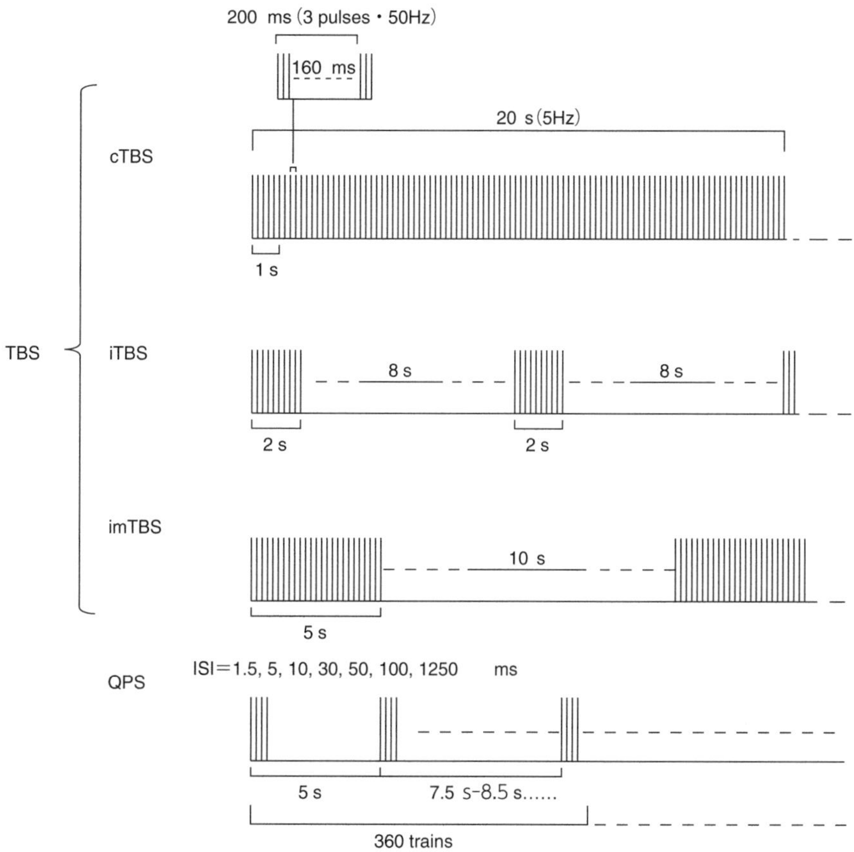

Fig. 8.3 Schematic diagram of patterned TMS

Each patient received a 15-day treatment session consisting of (1) transcranial stimulation to the nonlesional hemisphere with 2400 pulses (80 % of the motor threshold of the first dorsal interosseous muscles at rest) via cTBS, which continuously provides three repeated stimulations of 50 Hz at 5 Hz, (2) tailored occupational therapy for 120 minutes, and (3) self-exercise for 120 minutes. The upper limb function was evaluated twice using FMA and WMFT on the day of hospitalization and the day before discharge. The treatment and the study were approved as a clinical study by the Ethical Review Board at Shimizu Hospital, and the doctors obtained written consent from their patients.

This treatment protocol was accomplished without any adverse events in all the subjects. The change in FMA and WMFT before and after treatment suggested the improvement of the upper limb motor function. While it has already been reported that conducting NEURO-15 in poststroke patients with hemiparesis can improve the upper limb function, a similar result was obtained when conducting TBS in this study. One of the advantages of TBS is that the stimulation lasts only 3 minutes and both patient's and medical staff's burden can be reduced. Future studies on the long-run effect are required, however; we believe that the combination protocol of theta burst consecutive magnetic stimulation, which is our idea, and intensive occupational therapy can be a new treatment for upper limb hemiparesis in poststroke patients [17].

B. What Is Bihemispheric rTMS?

Here we present previous research in which both conventional low-frequency and high-frequency rTMS were applied to both of the hemispheres. When rTMS is used for therapeutic purposes, methods that directly apply high-frequency rTMS to the affected hemisphere could take in a compensatory role, and methods that apply low-frequency rTMS to the nonlesional hemisphere weaken the interhemispheric inhibition of the affected hemisphere, thus trying to indirectly activate sites that can compensate for lost functions by releasing them from interhemispheric inhibition.

Although various studies have been conducted to examine the merits and demerits of these two approaches, it is still not clear which is superior; both high-frequency rTMS and low-frequency rTMS have merits and demerits. Regardless of which approach is used, the application of rTMS induces neuroplasticity, and promotes the functional recovery of the paralyzed hand of stroke patients. On the grounds of the interhemispheric competition model of poststroke patients, we believe that by applying high-frequency rTMS to the affected hemisphere in addition to low-frequency rTMS to the nonlesional hemisphere greater improvement might be achieved than with unilateral rTMS alone.

There is no report on the combined application of high-frequency and low-frequency rTMS for therapeutic purposes in poststroke patients in combination with intensive rehabilitation on consecutive days. Therefore, we present here a research paper in which we determined the safety of 10-Hz high-frequency rTMS and its efficacy in the treatment of poststroke patients with upper limb hemiparesis when applied to the affected hemisphere in addition to NEURO-15, which is a combination of low-frequency rTMS and intensive rehabilitation and was used as basic treatment [18].

This study included eight poststroke patients with upper limb hemiparesis who were hospitalized at our department between September 17 and December 17 in 2011 and received high-frequency rTMS (10 Hz) to the affected hemisphere + NEURO-15, and whose BRS were stage III to V for both upper limb and hand-finger (mean age: 62.8 ± 4.9 years old, mean time after stroke: 84.3 ± 87.2 months, type of stroke: four intracerebral hemorrhage, four cerebral infarction). The eligibility criteria were similar to those for NEURO-15 shown in Chap. 2 (p. 21).

All eight patients were treated as follows: (i) the affected and unaffected hemispheres were stimulated alternatively with a total of 4000 pulses/day, namely, 2000 pulses each of low-frequency (1 Hz) stimulation to the unaffected hemisphere and high-frequency (10-Hz) stimulation to the affected hemisphere (10 Hz for

Table 8.4 Hospitalization schedule for bihemispheric rTMS[a]

	Day 1	Day 2	Day 3–7	Day 8	Day 10–13	Day 14	Day 15
Morning	Admission		Bihemispheric rTMS (40 minutes)		Bihemispheric rTMS (40 minutes)	Bihemispheric rTMS (40 minutes)	Discharge
		Low-freq. rTMS (20 minutes)	One-to-one OT (80 minutes)	Low-freq. rTMS (20 minutes)	One-to-one OT (80 minutes)	One-to-one OT (40 minutes)	
		Self-exercise (60 minutes)	Self-exercise (60 minutes)	Self-exercise (60 minutes)	Self-exercise (60 minutes)	Self-exercise (60 minutes)	
Afternoon	Evaluation of upper limb function	One-to-one OT (60 minutes)	One-to-one OT (40 minutes)	One-to-one OT (60 minutes)	One-to-one OT (40 minutes)	Evaluation of upper limb function	
		Self-exercise (60 minutes)	Self-exercise (60 minutes)	Self-exercise (60 minutes)	Self-exercise (60 minutes)		

[a]Complete rest on Day 9

5 seconds, followed by 1 Hz for 50 seconds, and this cycle was repeated 40 times). Moreover, during the 15-day hospitalization period daily treatment sessions consisting of (ii) one-to-one OT 6 units/day (40 minutes × 3) and (iii) self-exercise 120 minutes/day were conducted. The hospitalization schedule of this therapy is shown in Table 8.4.

The stimulation site and the intensity of low-frequency rTMS were determined on the day of admission. The stimulation site was set as the hand-finger areas in the primary motor cortex of the unaffected hemisphere, and the intensity of stimulation was set at 90 % of the minimum stimulation intensity that induces motor evoked potentials (MEPs) of maximum peak-to-peak amplitude in the abductor pollicis brevis muscle of the nonparalyzed upper limb. Low-frequency rTMS was applied by use of MagPro R30 and figure-8 coil (both manufactured by MagVenture). Actual treatment by bihemispheric rTMS in a clinical setting is shown in Fig. 8.4. Moreover, motor function of the upper limb was evaluated by use of FMA, WMFT, and MAS on the day of admission and discharge.

As a result, this treatment protocol was completed in all patients without observing any adverse events. Changes in FMA, WMFT, and MAS before and after treatment suggested an improvement in motor function of the upper limb in all patients (Table 8.5). Moreover, a statistically significant improvement was observed in the results of FMA, WMFT, and MAS before and after treatment (Table 8.6).

In this treatment, the first and strong approach in which consecutive rTMS is given alternatively to both hemispheres for 11 days in combination with intensive rehabilitation can lead to a long-term effect of motor function improvement and functional reorganization in a use-dependent manner. We believe that simultaneous stimulation with low- and high-frequency rTMS combined with intensive OT may become a new therapeutic approach for the treatment of poststroke upper limb hemiparesis [18].

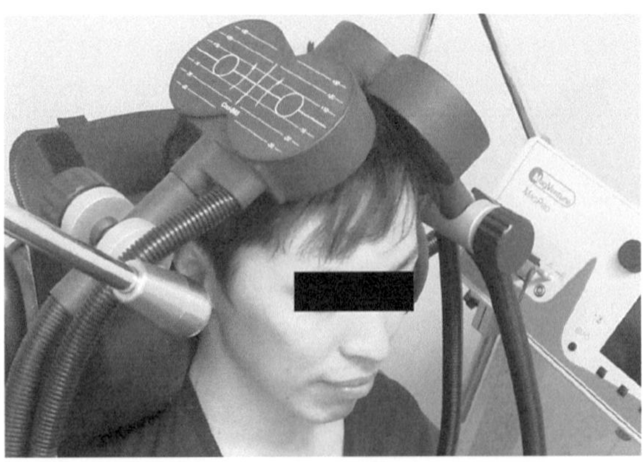

Fig. 8.4 Bihemispheric rTMS in a clinical setting

Table 8.5 Motor function evaluation results

			WMFT				MAS					
	FMA for upper limb		Performance time of 15 tasks (seconds)		FAS		Finger flexor muscle group		Wrist flexor muscle group		Elbow flexor muscle group	
Patient no.	Pre-treatment	Post-treatment	Pre-treatment	Post-treatment	Pre-treatment	Post-treatment	Pre-treatment	Post-treatment	Pre-treatment	Post-treatment	Pre-treatment	Post-treatment
1	46	57	573.6	329.1	37	47	3	1	1.5	0	2	1.5
2	37	38	884.2	388.8	31	45	2	1	1.5	0	1.5	1
3	47	56	59.7	39.8	48	59	1.5	1	1.5	0	0	0
4	54	63	197.6	176.5	57	66	1.5	0	1.5	1	1	0
5	49	52	1213.0	977.4	28	31	1	0	2	1.5	1	0
6	25	39	782.3	659.9	33	35	1.5	1	1.5	0	1.5	1
7	27	41	857.0	135.2	32	46	1	0	1	0	1	1
8	44	53	522.49	186.81	41	49	1	0	1	0	1.5	1

Table 8.6 Statistical data of the results of motor function evaluation[a]

Evaluation method	Outcome measure	Pre-treatment	Post-treatment	*P* value
BRS	Upper limb	3.4±0.7	3.5±0.8	N.S
	Hand-fingers	4.0±0.5	4.4±0.7	N.S
MAS	Elbow flexor muscle group	1.2±0.6	0.7±0.6	<0.05
	Wrist flexor muscle group	1.4±0.3	0.3±0.6	<0.05
	Finger flexor muscle group	1.6±0.7	0.5±0.5	<0.05
	Total score	41.1±10.5	49.9±9.4	<0.05
FMA	Evaluation item A	24.8±6.1	28.0±4.9	N.S
	Evaluation item B	5.1±1.7	7.8±1.5	<0.05
	Evaluation item C	8.6±3.5	11.1±3.7	<0.05
	Evaluation item D	2.6±1.6	3.0±1.7	N.S
WMFT	Performance time for 15 tasks (seconds)	636.2±379.1	361.7±313.9	<0.05
	Natural logarithm of mean performance time	3.5±1.0	2.8±1.0	<0.05

[a]All evaluation results are expressed as mean±SD

References

1. Scott AB. Botulinum toxin injection into extra-ocular muscles as an alternative to strabismus surgery. Ophthalmology. 1980;87:1044–9.
2. Ko CP. Do nerve terminal sprouts contribute to functional recovery from botulinum neurotoxin A? J Physiol. 2008;586:3021.
3. Caty GD, Detrembleur C, Bleyenheuft C, et al. Effect of upper limb botulinum toxin injections on impairment, activity, participation, and quality of life among stroke patients. Stroke. 2009;40:2589–91.
4. Watkins CL, Leathley MJ, Gregson JM, et al. Prevalence of spasticity post stroke. Clin Rehabil. 2002;16:515–22.
5. Ward AB, Turner-Stokes L. The management of adults with spasticity using botulinum toxin; a guide to clinical practice. London: Radius Healthcare; 2001.
6. Sheehan G, Lannin NA, Turner-Stokes L, et al. Botulinum toxin assessment, intervention and after-care for upper limb hypertonicity in adults: international consensus statement. Eur J Neurol. 2010;17 Suppl 2:74–93.
7. Kakuda W, Abo M, Momosaki R, et al. Combined therapeutic application of botulinum toxin type A, low-frequency rTMS, and intensive occupational therapy for post-stroke spastic upper limb hemiparesis. Eur J Phys Rehabil Med. 2011;48:47–55.
8. Wassermann EM. Risk and safety of repetitive transcranial magnetic stimulation: report and suggested guidelines from the international workshop on the safety of repetitive transcranial magnetic stimulation, June 5–7, 1996. Electroencephalogr Clin Neurophysiol. 1998;108:1–16.
9. Naoki Yamada, Wataru Kakuda, Takahiro Kondo, et al. Local muscle injection of botulinum toxin type A synergistically improves the beneficial effects of repetitive transcranial magnetic stimulation and intensive occupational therapy in post-stroke patients with spastic upper limb hemiparesis. Eur Neurol. 2014. doi:10.1159/000365005.
10. Hikosaka O, Takikawa Y, Kawgoe R. Role of the basal ganglia in the control of purposive saccadic eye movements. Physiol Rev. 2000;80:954–78.

11. Schultz W. Predictive reward signal of dopamine neurons. J Neurophysiol. 1998;80:1–27.
12. Scheidtmann K, Fries W, Müller F, et al. Effect of levodopa in combination with physiotherapy on functional motor recovery after stroke: a prospective, randomised, double-blind study. Lancet. 2001;358:787–90.
13. Kakuda W, Abo M, Kobayashi K, et al. Combination treatment of low-frequency rTMS and occupational therapy with levodopa administration; an intensive neurorehabilitative approach for upper limb hemiparesis after stroke. Int J Neurosci. 2011;121:373–8.
14. Rossi S, Hallett M, Rossini PM, et al. Safety, ethical considerations, and application guidelines for the use of transcranial magnetic stimulation in clinical practice and research. Clin Neurophysiol. 2009;120:2008–39.
15. Hamada M, Ugawa Y, Tsuji S. High-frequency rTMS over the supplementary motor area improves bradykinesia in Parkinson's disease; subanalysis of double-blind sham-controlled study. J Neurol Sci. 2009;287:143–6.
16. Huang YZ, Edwards MJ, Rounis E, et al. Theta burst stimulation of the human motor cortex. Neuron. 2005;45:201–6.
17. Yamada N, Kakuda W, Kondo T, et al. Continuous theta-burst stimulation combined with occupational therapy for upper limb hemiparesis after stroke: a preliminary study. Acta Neurol Belg. 3 Apr 2014 [Epub ahead of print].
18. Yamada N, Kakuda W, Kondo T, et al. Bihemispheric repetitive transcranial magnetic stimulation combined with intensive occupational therapy for upper limb hemiparesis after stroke; a preliminary study. Int J Rehabil Res. 2013;36:323–9.

Index

M. Abo, W. Kakuda, *Rehabilitation with rTMS*,
DOI 10.1007/978-3-319-20982-1